Student's Companion

Documentation and Pharmaceutical Regulatory Writing for Students and Practitioners

RXpert SERIES

Student's Companion

Documentation and Pharmaceutical Regulatory Writing for Students and Practitioners

Ajay G. Pise
M. Pharm, Ph. D.
Associate Professor,
Dadasaheb Balpande College of Pharmacy,
Besa, Nagpur,
Maharashtra – 440037.

Sandhya M. Bagde
M. Pharm, (Ph. D.),
Assistant Professor,
Dadasaheb Balpande College of Pharmacy,
Besa, Nagpur,
Maharashtra – 440037.

Ketki S. Ande
M. Pharm,
Regulatory Affairs Officer,
Sun Pharma, Vadodara,
Gujarat.

PharmaMed Press
An imprint of BSP Books Pvt. Ltd.
4-4-309/316, Giriraj Lane,
Sultan Bazar, Hyderabad - 500 095.

Documentation and Pharmaceutical Regulatory Writing for Students and Practitioners
by **Ajay G. Pise, Sandhya M. Bagde and Ketki S. Ande**

Disclaimer: The author and publishers have taken due care to provide authentic, reliable and up-to-date information related to the subject. However, neither the author nor the publisher shall be responsible for any liability for any damage caused because of the use of this book. The respective users must check the accuracy from other sources too.

Published by

PharmaMed Press ™
An imprint of BSP Books Pvt. Ltd.
4-4-309/316, Giriraj Lane, Sultan Bazar, Hyderabad - 500 095.
Phone: 040-23445688; Fax: 91+40-23445611
E-mail: info@pharmamedpress.net
www.bspbooks.net/www.pharmamedpress.net

ISBN: 978-93-49562-47-9 (Hardback)

CHAPTER 1

Documentation in Pharmaceutical Industry

Exploratory Product Development Brief (EPDB) for Drug Substance and Drug product

Numerous organizations are encountering an atmosphere that is marked by uncertainty, fast-changing trends, and growing complexity. In such an environment, where many variables are unknown and in flux, the conventional approach to product development cannot reliably identify new types of risk. It is not feasible to fully define a product before commencing development. If companies try to adhere to a traditional phased-and-gated process in a dynamic environment, the product development team is likely to struggle with managing the scope, timeline, and budget that were established at the outset. As a result, changes to product requirements, unexpected issues, rework, schedule delays, budget overruns, and commercial disappointment are all common outcomes. The product development team requires an approach that enables them to adapt to changes in customer needs, markets, competition, technology, and other factors.

ExPD presents a fresh method for developing products by utilizing a two-pronged solution:

1. Treating product development from a comprehensive systems perspective and
2. Fundamentally redesigning the development process to minimize project uncertainties and risk.

ExPD deviates from the conventional phased-and-gated process by fundamentally rethinking the development process to reduce uncertainties and risks. It is an adaptive approach that responds rapidly to changes in internal and external factors. This process enables project teams to identify, evaluate, and prioritize uncertainties and risks throughout a project. The team can then determine how and when to address the uncertainty or when it is appropriate to terminate a project.

Process Structure

ExPD is a holistic and integrated approach that consists of two primary components. According to Drotar and Morrissey, product development is a complex process that must be managed as a comprehensive system, incorporating critical elements such as strategy, portfolio management, organization/teams/culture, metrics, market/customer understanding, and process.

The first aspect of ExPD involves adopting a system-level perspective that integrates these essential components and recognizes their interrelationships. This approach enables the product development team to assess the impact of decisions and changes on the entire development process. The second component of ExPD involves redesigning the product development process to minimize uncertainties and risks by addressing the critical elements identified in the first component. By leveraging this two-pronged approach, ExPD offers a comprehensive and adaptable framework for product development that can effectively respond to the dynamic and constantly evolving nature of modern business environments.

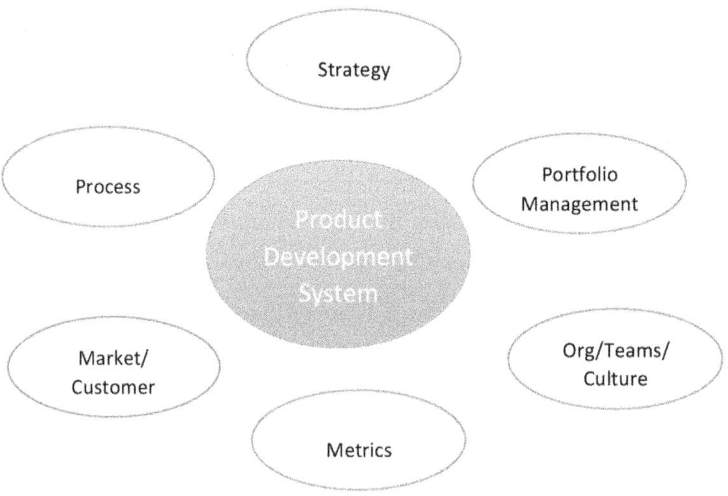

Figure 1.1 Exploratory product development system.

The two-pronged approach of exploratory product development differs from the traditional phase-gate process in that it involves a fundamental redesign of the product development process with a focus on reducing uncertainty and risk. Unlike the traditional approach, ExPD includes three interrelated segments in its process that work together to achieve this objective.

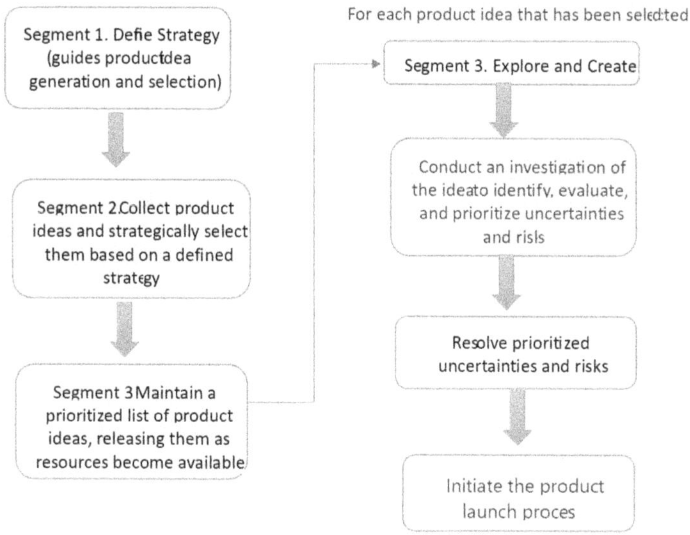

Figure 1.2 The three segments of exploratory product development.

1. **Strategy**

   In the ExPD process, strategy is a critical component and is considered essential to achieving success in product development. ExPD incorporates a strategic framework that provides direction for strategy development in stable, moderately dynamic, or highly dynamic environments. This framework ensures that the enterprise, business unit, and product categories are all aligned with the strategic goals of the organization. Strategy also plays a pivotal role in guiding the product idea generation and selection process, ensuring that the product development efforts are focused on meeting strategic objectives. Therefore, in the ExPD approach, strategy is integrated into every stage of the product development process to ensure that it is aligned with the overall business strategy and goals.

2. **Idea Generation and Selection**

   In the ExPD process, the goal of idea generation and selection is to generate a pool of new product ideas and evaluate them using the strategic framework. Once a promising product idea is identified, whether generated internally or externally, it is prioritized among other competing ideas and allocated resources before being assigned to a product team. The ExPD process includes a prioritization valve that allows for the prioritization of product ideas, taking into account the available resources and adjusting the flow of projects throughout the process. The prioritization valve helps illustrate the process of turning ideas on and off based on available resources, ensuring that the most promising ideas are given priority and that the product development process remains aligned with the company's strategic goals.

3. **Explore and Create**

   In the Explore and Create stage of ExPD, the product undergoes an Investigate phase where a cross-functional team identifies, evaluates, and prioritizes product uncertainties and risks. Based on this evaluation, the organization determines which products will be released into a resolution loop, where the product team focuses on reducing and resolving the prioritized uncertainties and risks. Once a product enters the resolution loop, the team uses a fast iterative/sprint approach to development, involving four key stages: Design, Build, Execute, and Learn (as shown in Figure 3). The resolution loop is designed to be adaptable to real-time learnings and changes in the environment.

   During the resolution loop, the product team not only works to resolve the most impactful uncertainties and risks, but also strives to develop a finished product that can be released to the market. By using a fast iterative/sprint approach, the team can continuously incorporate feedback and adapt to changing customer needs and market trends, ensuring that the final product is optimized for success in the market.

Product Development Plan (PDP)

The process of developing and launching a new product involves multiple stages, including strategizing, organizing, generating concepts, creating and evaluating product and marketing plans, and ultimately bringing the product to market. This process is crucial for companies looking to achieve significant growth, as new and innovative products are often the key driver of growth.

Product Development Report

A product development report is a document that outlines the various stages of a product's development, from conception to launch. The report typically includes information on the product's market research, design, testing, manufacturing, and marketing strategies. It is a critical document that provides an overview of the entire product development process, which can be used to assess the product's viability, profitability, and success.

Here are some key sections that are typically included in a product development report:

1. ***Executive Summary***: This section provides a brief overview of the product, the market opportunity it addresses, and the key findings of the report.

2. ***Market Research***: This section outlines the market research conducted to identify the target market, customer needs, and preferences, and the competitive landscape.
3. ***Design***: This section discusses the product design, including the design process, key features and functionalities, and the product's technical specifications.
4. ***Testing***: This section covers the testing and validation process, including the different types of testing performed, the results, and any changes made to the product based on feedback.
5. ***Manufacturing***: This section details the manufacturing process, including the materials used, the production process, quality control measures, and any challenges encountered.
6. ***Marketing Strategy***: This section outlines the marketing strategy for the product, including the target audience, pricing strategy, distribution channels, and promotional activities.
7. ***Financial Projections***: This section includes financial projections for the product, including revenue, expenses, and profit margins.
8. ***Conclusion***: This section summarizes the key findings of the report and provides recommendations for the next steps in the product development process.

Overall, a product development report serves as a comprehensive document that provides an overview of the entire product development process. It is a critical tool for assessing the viability and success of a product and can be used to make informed decisions about future product development efforts.

MASTER FORMULA RECORD

The Master Formula Record (MFR) is a crucial document for pharmaceutical products, containing comprehensive information about the manufacturing process. It is typically created by the company's research and development team and serves as a reference standard for preparing the batch manufacturing record (BMR) by manufacturing units. In addition, the MFR may also be referred to as the Master Manufacturing Record or Master Production Record.

"A document or set of documents specifying the starting materials with their quantities and the packaging materials, together with a description of the procedures and precautions required to produce a specified quantity of a finished product as well as the processing instructions, including the in-process controls."

To ensure consistency in each batch manufacturing, it is necessary to have Master Formula records for all manufacturing procedures of each product and batch size. These records are prepared and endorsed by competent technical staff, such as the head of production and quality control. MFR serves as a reference standard for the preparation of batch manufacturing records (BMR) by manufacturing units. Having MFR is crucial in maintaining the quality and consistency of the product throughout its manufacturing process.

MFR should include:

Product Details:

- Name, logo and address of the manufacturing company.
- Dosage form name.
- Brand name.
- Generic name.
- Product code
- Label the claim of all ingredients
- Product description
- Batch size
- Pack size and packing style
- Shelf life
- Storage conditions
- MFR number and date
- Supersede MFR number and date
- Effective batch number
- Authorization by the production and quality assurance head

Procedure to prepare a Master Formula Record:

A Master Formula Record can be created by experienced and qualified personnel such as manufacturing chemists or analytical chemists, or by using the batch manufacturing record of a previous batch size. It is essential to follow the Master Formula Record at all stages of production, and it is transferred from previous staff to new staff as a standard document for processing each batch. The Master Formula Record serves as a reference standard for creating a Batch Manufacturing Record and plays a critical role in ensuring consistency across batches.

SOP for preparation of the Master Formula Record:

RESPONSIBLE DEPARTMENTS:

Primary Responsibility: F&D and Production Department

Secondary Responsibility: Quality Assurance Department

ACCOUNTABILITY:

Head-Quality Assurance shall be responsible for the implementation of SOP.

STEPS TO PREPARE A MASTER FORMULA RECORD:

1. The Production Department in association with F&D (Formulation and Development) shall prepare the MFR.
2. The MFR should be prepared as per the format attached to the SOP.
3. The MFR should be divided into two parts - Packaging and Manufacturing parts.
4. The first page of both sections should have the following details:
   - Name, address, and logo of the company
   - Dosage form name
   - Brand name
   - Generic name
   - Product code
   - Label claim: This should include all ingredients and text included in product permission.
   - Product Description
   - Batch size
   - Pack size
   - Shelf life
   - Storage conditions
   - Drug Schedule: Whether Schedule H or Schedule G drug.
   - Superseded Master card number and date
   - Present Master card number and date
   - Present Master card effective batch number
   - Reference of changed control number
5. The MFR should be authorized by all the responsible members.
6. The secondary page of the manufacturing section should include process steps to be monitored.
7. Subsequent pages should include the processes to be monitored in a stage-wise movement of material in the form of a flow chart.
8. The list of equipment, machines, and utensils to be used should be described.
9. The subsequent page should include any special precautions to be taken for the product during manufacturing and packing. The same page should also include the Batch Manufacturing Formula.

10. The Batch Formula should have the following columns:
    - Serial number
    - Name of ingredients
    - Reference of specifications of ingredients
    - Quantity to be added (in mg/ml or per tablet or per capsule or per gm, as the case may be)
    - Overages to be added (in %)
    - Quantity to be added per batch or per lot
11. Calculation steps should be given for every active material, ensuring that the active material shall be compensated for assay values less than 100%, which could be due to less potency or higher moisture content.

The MFR should also include the testing requirements for raw materials, intermediate products, and finished products, along with their specifications and acceptable limits. Any special instructions for sampling and testing of materials should be mentioned. The MFR should also include the specifications for environmental controls, such as temperature and humidity, during the manufacturing process. Document should specify the cleaning procedures and acceptance criteria for equipment and facilities. MFR should also include the specifications for labeling and storage of finished products. The document should mention any precautions or warnings that need to be taken during the manufacturing process to ensure the safety of personnel and the environment. Finally, the MFR should be reviewed and approved by authorized personnel before being implemented.

BATCH MANUFACTURING RECORD

A batch manufacturing record should be prepared for each intermediate or API/formulation, containing complete information on its manufacturing and quality control. The batch manufacturing record should be carefully reviewed before issuance to ensure that it is the correct version and accurately reproduces the master production instruction. Before beginning any manufacturing operations, a check must be conducted and recorded to confirm that the equipment and workspace are clear of any previous products, documents, or materials not required for the current process and that the equipment is clean and suitable for use. Each batch record should be assigned a unique identification number, and dated and signed at the time of issuance.

The "Batch Manufacturing Record" is an important document for ensuring the quality and compliance of the manufacturing process. It is a record that contains all the information related to the manufacture of a specific batch or lot of a product, including the ingredients used, manufacturing steps, in-process tests and results, and any deviations from the standard operating procedures. The BMR provides complete traceability of the product from the raw materials to the finished product and is a critical tool for ensuring consistency and quality throughout the manufacturing process.

These are all important pieces of information that should be included in the Batch Manufacturing Record (BMR).

In addition to these, it is important to note that the BMR should also include details on the specific procedures followed for each step in the manufacturing process, including any safety precautions or measures taken. It should also include information on any environmental conditions or controls necessary for the production process, such as temperature, humidity, or air pressure.

Finally, the BMR must be reviewed and approved by a designated quality control unit before the release of the batch for distribution. This helps ensure that all necessary steps have been followed and documented and that the final product meets all specifications and requirements.

Responsibility:

Primary: Officer–QA / Officer–QC/ Officer-Production

Secondary: Manager-QA/ Manager- QC/ Manager- Production

Issue of batch manufacturing record (by Quality Assurance)

1. Based on Production planning, the production manager shall decide on the product and the number of batches to be produced in the month.
2. The production supervisor shall raise the requisition for the batches to be taken for the week and forward it to Quality Assurance.
3. On receipt of Batch Manufacturing Record issue requisition QA personnel will verify the details entered in the requisition form.
4. A photocopy of the MASTER COPY of the required Product Batch Manufacturing Record will be taken.
5. All the pages of the photocopied sheet of the Product Batch Manufacturing Record shall be signed and dated by QA Personnel.
6. Check for the correctness of the Batch number by verifying the BMR register.
7. Enter the details of Date, Product, Batch No, Batch size, Manufacturing Date, Expiry Date, and issued by details in the BMR register.
8. Check and allot expiry date by referring to the master list of product shelf life.
9. Enter batch no. On all the pages of the BMR and get it authorized by QA manager or in the absence by QA executive or QA officer.
10. Insert the signed batch record in a BMR cover and enter the details of the product name, batch number, and batch size. Manufacturing date and expiry date.

11. The batch record along with the batch record register shall be sent to production, the production person receiving the batch record should sign on the batch record register to acknowledge the receipt of the batch record.
12. QA person who has issued Batch Record shall sign the "issued by" on the batch record issue requisition sheet and file the same for future reference.
13. Before issuing the batch record, QA personnel should ensure that all necessary documentation, such as analytical reports and quality control test results, are available and reviewed for each batch.
14. If any discrepancies or deviations are found, they should be recorded in the batch record and investigated before issuing the record.
15. The batch record should be issued to the production department promptly to ensure that production activities can begin as scheduled.
16. All batch records should be stored in a secure location with proper traceability and retrievability.
17. The batch record issue process should be periodically reviewed and updated as necessary to ensure continued effectiveness.

Entry of Batch Manufacturing Records (By Production Personnel)

1. The first step in the entry of Batch Manufacturing Records (BMR) by Production Personnel is for the Production Manager or Deputy Production Manager to check the BMR and sign on the first page to indicate that they have reviewed it. This ensures that there is a level of oversight and accountability in the production process.
2. The calculation sheet is forwarded to the stores' department so that the relevant analytical reference (AR) numbers, quantity, and assay values can be entered. This information is necessary for tracking the usage of raw materials and intermediates during the manufacturing process. The stores department is responsible for maintaining the inventory of all the raw materials, intermediates, and other supplies required for manufacturing. They update the inventory records after the entry of the relevant information in the calculation sheet.
3. It appears that after a relevant entry is made, a sheet is forwarded to the production department. In the production department, a production chemist fills in equipment status details for each piece of equipment, including the line clearance status and ECR number.
4. Where the operator fills out a form for the specific process to be carried out on a particular reactor. The form requires the starting and ending time of the process to be entered and for the operator to sign it. The form is then checked by an in-charge.

5. After completion of every reaction in each of the particular reactors, the intermediate product is sent to the QC (Quality Control) Lab for checking. The purpose of sending the intermediate product to the QC Lab is to ensure that the reaction has been completed as intended and that the product meets the necessary quality standards. The QC Lab will typically check the product for various parameters, such as the level of completion of the reaction, the impurities present in the product, and the level of moisture or other contaminants (which is usually measured by LOD or Loss on Drying).
6. After the final product is obtained, a request is sent to the QC (Quality Control) department for a complete analysis of the product. Once the analysis is complete, the QC department will generate an analytical report, which details the results of the analysis and provides information on the quality and specifications of the product. This report is then sent back to the manufacturing department, where it is reviewed to ensure that the product meets all of the necessary requirements.
7. In the manufacturing process, where all remaining entries are filled out and all analytical reports are attached.
8. The BMR (Batch Manufacturing Record) is sent to the QA (Quality Assurance) department for review.

Review and Control of Batch Manufacturing Records (by Quality Assurance)

1. The QA (Quality Assurance) department checks the batch number. The batch number is a unique identifier assigned to each batch of product that is manufactured. It is used to track the product throughout its lifecycle, from manufacturing to distribution and sale. The purpose of checking the batch number is to ensure that the correct product has been manufactured and that it meets all of the necessary quality standards and specifications.
2. Review the analytical report of all raw materials attached with BMR and check the A.R. No. This step ensures that all raw materials used in the manufacturing process were of the appropriate quality and that the analytical testing was performed according to the approved procedures.
3. Review the Equipment Cleaning Record for each piece of equipment and the relevance of line clearance by QC. This step ensures that all equipment used in the manufacturing process was properly cleaned and that there was no cross-contamination between different batches of product.
4. Review the deviation in the process which is predefined. This step involves reviewing any deviations or exceptions that occurred during the manufacturing process and ensuring that they were properly documented and addressed.

5. If any deviation is present, change the deviation report of the process. Review the report of change in deviation and its significance in the process. This step involves reviewing any changes made to the manufacturing process as a result of deviations or exceptions and ensuring that they were properly documented and approved.
6. Check the quantity of solvent recovered in the process. Recovery should be proper and complete. This step ensures that all solvents used in the manufacturing process were properly recovered and that there was no waste or loss of materials.
7. Wet material packing records should be reviewed. This step involves reviewing the records of the packing of wet materials to ensure that they were properly packaged and labeled.
8. The drying record as well as the dry material packing record should be checked and reviewed. This step involves reviewing the records of the drying process and the packing of dry materials to ensure that they were properly dried, packaged, and labeled.
9. Check the analytical report of the finished product generated by QC department. This step involves reviewing the final analytical report of the finished product to ensure that it meets all of the necessary quality standards and specifications.
10. Finally, attach the review report with a specific number given by the QA department duly dated and signed by the QA manager. This step involves documenting all of the reviews and approvals that were performed during the manufacturing process.
11. If everything is fine, then pass the batch and allow it for dispatch. This step involves releasing the batch for distribution and sale.
12. Send this record to the safe custody of the Quality Assurance department. This step involves storing the BMR and all associated documentation in a safe and secure location for future reference.
13. If anybody needs a copy of the BMR, it should be given as a control copy with the permission of the QA manager. This step ensures that access to the BMR and associated documentation is controlled and limited to authorized personnel.
14. Every BMR should be saved for five years from manufacturing and after that, it should be destroyed as per SOP. This step ensures that all documentation related to the manufacturing process is properly stored and disposed of in accordance with company policies and regulatory requirements.

Batch Manufacturing Record Attachments Responsibility:

Primary: Production Chemist.

Secondary: Production Officer.

These attachments provide a complete record of the manufacturing process, ensuring traceability and accountability for the final product. It is important to ensure that all necessary attachments are included before submitting the BMR to the Quality Assurance department.

1. Analytical report of raw materials
2. Analytical report of the finished product
3. Process validation report (if applicable)
4. Stability study report (if applicable)
5. Change control request (if any changes were made during the manufacturing process)
6. Batch release certificate signed by the Quality Assurance department.

BATCH PACKING RECORD

A Batch Packing Record (BPR) is a document that provides instructions and records for the packing of a specific batch of a product. It contains detailed information about the packaging process, including the materials and equipment used, the batch number, the quantity of product being packed, and the packaging instructions.

The following information is typically included in a Batch Packing Record:

1. Batch number and product code
2. Date of packing and name of the person responsible
3. Packaging instructions, including the type and size of packaging material, label information, and special instructions
4. Equipment and tools used for packing
5. Verification of packaging materials and equipment, including their condition and suitability for use
6. Record of quantity of product packed
7. Record of any deviations or incidents that occurred during the packing process
8. Signatures and dates of personnel involved in the packing process
9. In-process test results and any associated documentation.

The Batch Packing Record is an essential document for ensuring the consistency and quality of the final packaged product. It is used by the Quality Assurance department to verify that the product has been packed according to the approved specifications and that all relevant documentation has been completed and reviewed.

To ensure accurate and reliable packaging of each batch or part batch, it is essential to maintain a batch packaging record. This record should be created based on the relevant parts of the packaging instructions. At every stage of the packaging process, the responsible person should record the actions taken, along with the date and their signature or electronic password.

The information to be documented includes the product name, batch number, and quantity of bulk product to be packed, as well as the planned and actual quantities of the finished product obtained. The record should also include details of the packaging operations, equipment used, in-process checks, and any deviation from the packaging instructions with appropriate authorization. Finally, the record should provide a reconciliation of the quantities of printed packaging materials and bulk products issued, used, destroyed, or returned to stock.

(a) Record the name of the product, its batch number, the quantity of bulk product to be packed, the planned quantity of finished product to be obtained, the actual quantity obtained, and the reconciliation.

(b) Note down the date(s) and time(s) of the packaging operations.

(c) Identify the name of the person responsible for carrying out the packaging operation.

(d) Record the initials of the operators with different roles and responsibilities.

(e) Document the checks performed for identity and conformity with the packaging instructions, including the results of in-process controls.

(f) The batch packaging record should include details of all packaging operations performed, including the equipment and packaging lines used. In cases where the product needs to be kept unpacked or returned to storage, clear instructions should be included in the record.

(g) Wherever possible, samples of the printed packaging materials used should be included in the record. These should bear the batch number, expiry date, and any additional overprinting.

(h) Any special problems encountered during the packaging process should be noted in the record. This includes any deviations from the packaging instructions, which must be authorized in writing by an appropriate person.

(i) The record should include the quantities and reference numbers or identification of all printed packaging materials and bulk products that were issued, used, destroyed, or returned to stock. These quantities should permit an adequate reconciliation of the product obtained.

DOCUMENTATION

Documentation is an essential part of any quality assurance system, and it serves as a record of the manufacturing process, ensuring that the final product meets the required standards. Clear and accurate documentation helps to prevent errors and enables the tracing of the batch history. Manufacturing specifications, formulae, instructions, procedures, and records must be free from errors and available in written form to ensure that the process is reproducible and consistent. Good documentation practices are critical for ensuring product quality, safety, and efficacy, and they are a key element of Good Manufacturing Practices (GMP) regulations.

The purpose of documentation in pharmaceutical manufacturing includes:

1. ***Defining specifications and procedures*:** Documentation provides clear and detailed instructions for all materials and methods of manufacture and control. This ensures that processes are consistent, reproducible, and meet quality standards.
2. ***Ensuring personnel are informed*:** Documentation ensures that all personnel involved in the manufacturing process understand their roles and responsibilities, and know what actions to take at each step.
3. ***Ensuring product release*:** Documentation provides the necessary information for authorized persons to decide whether or not to release a batch of a drug for sale, based on the results of quality assurance checks.
4. ***Providing traceability and audit trail*:** Documentation creates a record of all activities, providing an audit trail and traceability. This allows for investigations and helps identify the root cause of any issues that may arise.
5. ***Facilitating validation, review, and statistical analysis*:** Documentation provides the data needed for validation, review, and statistical analysis, which are essential components of quality assurance in the pharmaceutical industry.

PACKAGING INSTRUCTION

Packaging instructions are formal documents that must be approved for each product pack size and type. These instructions should contain or reference the following information:

1. The product name.
2. A description of its pharmaceutical form, strength, and, if applicable, method of application.
3. The pack size is expressed as the number, weight, or volume of the product in the final container.
4. A complete list of all packaging materials required for standard batch size, including quantities, sizes, and types, with codes or reference numbers linking to the specifications for each material.
5. If appropriate, an example or replica of relevant printed packaging materials and samples indicating where the batch number and expiry date are marked.
6. A meticulous inspection of the packaging area and equipment to ensure line clearance before starting operations.
7. A description of the packaging operation, including any significant subsidiary operations and equipment to be used.

8. Detailed in-process control instructions, including sampling and acceptance limits.

STERILE WATER FOR INJECTION

Sterile Water for Injection is a sterile and bacteria-free preparation of distilled water that does not contain any solutes. Its primary use is as a solvent or diluent for drugs or solutions that are suitable for intravenous or intramuscular administration. When used in this way, it provides hydration and facilitates drug delivery to the patient. It is typically the pharmacist who adds any required additives and relabels the container for use by the patient.

COMPONENTS OF BATCH PACKAGING RECORD FOR STERILE WATER FOR INJECTION

- Product name
- Batch number
- Formulation details
- Date, time, code number, and pack number
- Description of the packaging operation, including line clearance
- In-process checks performed during packaging
- Initials of the personnel responsible for the packaging checks

PACKAGING OPERATION

LINE CLEARANCE

Packaging line No	Previous Products
	Batch No

Sr.no	Activity	Removed checked	Done by	Checked by
1	Labeled vials, de-labeled vials, cartons, Insert, wrappers of the previous product/b.no on the table			
2	Labels, cartoons, and inserts of previous products near the labeling machine			
3	Waste from dustbins			
4	Rejected vials, labels, cartons, and inserts of the previous product/b.no for destruction			
5	Stamps removed from previous product /b.no			
6	Packed shippers shifted previous product/b.no to BSR 2			

DISTRIBUTION RECORDS

Distribution records must include the product name, strength, and dosage form, as well as the consignee's name and address, the shipment date and quantity, and the lot or control number of the drug product. Compressed medical gas products are exempt from the requirement of lot or control numbers in their distribution records.

The main purpose of these records is to provide sufficient data for contacting trade customers in case of a product recall. Assigning a lot number to each order is an effective way to achieve this goal. The recording of the dates, when a specific lot of product began and ended its distribution, can also be useful. This allows all customers who received the product between those dates to be identified and contacted.

There may be some overlap on the first and last days of distribution, as some customers may receive products from the previous or next lot. However, this should not compromise the recall effectiveness. Whatever system is used, it should allow for the reintroduction of returned goods into the distribution chain. Distribution records encompass a wide range of documentation, such as invoices, bills of lading, customers' receipts, and internal warehouse storage and inventory records. Not all documents need to include all the required information, and customer and product codes can be used as alternatives to names and addresses.

CERTIFICATE OF ANALYSIS (COA)

A Certificate of Analysis (COA) is a Quality Assurance document that verifies a regulated product's compliance with its specifications. It typically includes the test results obtained during quality control testing of a specific batch of the product. The company responsible for the material should prepare and issue the COA.

Purpose and Scope

The purpose of a Certificate of Analysis is to provide a report of analytical results for a specific batch of raw materials, components, APIs, finished products, or other similar items. It is typically issued by the company responsible for the material and includes actual results obtained from testing performed as part of quality control measures. The scope of a COA is limited to the specific batch of the product being analyzed.

The COA must be reviewed and approved by a designated representative of the testing site and must include the following information:

- Vendor or supplier details
- Product information, including name and strength
- Test results for the specific batch, including the name of the test, acceptance criteria, and the actual results obtained
- A statement indicating whether the product conforms to the specified requirements
- References to the method and specification documents used for the testing
- Information about the source of the data presented
- Approval and date of issuance
- Expiration date or retest information, if applicable.

The following information is required for a Certificate of Analysis (COA):

- Name and batch number of the product
- Manufacturer of the product
- The manufacturing date of the product
- Retest date of the product
- The expiry date of the product
- Transport instructions for the product
- Storage conditions for the product
- Content of reference substance in the product
- Note how the contents were calculated
- Any special handling requirements for the product
- Results for all required tests, including their specifications.

Certificate of Analysis: e-COA

The use of electronic Certificates of Analysis (e-COAs) is becoming increasingly common and is acceptable if appropriate controls are in place. To ensure the validity and accuracy of e-COAs, the following considerations should be met:

(a) Access to the computer system should be restricted to authorized personnel only. This includes limitations on data entry and editing, with user authentication through username and password. Additionally, the integrity and accuracy of the system should be confirmed during implementation and regularly checked thereafter.

(b) Data entered into the computer system should be time- and date-stamped, and accompanied by audit trails to track any changes made. If these criteria are met, electronically generated COAs can be considered valid. However, e-COAs must include contact information for the issuing entity.

The certificate should include:

- The name and address of the laboratory that conducted the tests.
- The registration number of the certificate of analysis.
- Details of the batch for which the certificate is issued, including the name, description (such as grade, quantity received, and type of container), and batch number used by the original manufacturer and repacker/trader. It should also include the date of manufacture and the expiry date or retest date.
- The date on which the batch was received for testing.
- A reference to the test procedure used, including the acceptance criteria (limits).
- The results of all tests performed on the batch, including numerical values and comparison with established acceptance criteria.
- Any additional test results obtained from samples taken as part of a periodic statistically based testing program.
- A statement indicating whether the batch met the requirements.
- The date or dates on which the tests were performed.
- The signature of the head of the laboratory or an authorized person.
- The name, address, telephone number, and fax number of the original manufacturer. If supplied by a repacker or trader, the certificate should also include their contact details and a reference to the original manufacturer.
- A statement of the expected conditions of shipping, packaging, storage, and distribution, which must be followed to maintain the validity of the certificate.
- If the sample was supplied by a repacker or trader, a copy of the certificate generated by the original manufacturer should also be included.

Model certificate of analysis for active pharmaceutical ingredients, excipients, and medicinal products

Registration number of sample or certificate: ____________________________

Name and address of laboratory testing the sample:

____

Sample information

Name of product (INN, brand name(s), etc.):

____

Dosage Form (if applicable):____________________________

Marketing authorization number(if applicable):______________________

Description (appearance of container and contents):

____

____

Batch number(s): ____________________________________

Conditions:__________________

Data received: ____________________

Date of manufacture: ____________________________________

Expiry date (for medicinal products) or retest date (for starting materials or excipients):____________________________

Name and address of original manufacturer:

Telephone:_______________ Fax:_____________

SITE MASTER FILE

The pharmaceutical manufacturer creates the Site Master File (SMF) to provide specific information about the quality management policies and activities, as well as the production and/or quality control operations carried out at the named site and any closely integrated operations at adjacent and nearby buildings. If only a part of a pharmaceutical operation is carried out on the site, the SMF should only describe those operations. When submitted to regulatory authorities, the SMF should provide information on the manufacturer's good manufacturing practices (GMP) related activities for the general supervision and efficient planning and undertaking of GMP inspections.

The SMF should contain adequate information but should not exceed 25-30 pages plus appendices. Simple plans, outline drawings or schematic layouts are preferred instead of narratives. The SMF, including appendices, should be easily readable when printed on A4 paper sheets. It should be a part of the documentation belonging to the quality management system of the manufacturer and kept updated accordingly. The SMF should have an edition number, an effective date, and a review date. It should be regularly reviewed to ensure it is up-to-date and representative of current activities.

Purpose

These explanatory notes are intended to assist pharmaceutical manufacturers in creating a Site Master File (SMF) that is relevant and helpful to regulatory authorities during Good Manufacturing Practice (GMP) inspections.

Scope

These guidelines are intended to assist manufacturers of medicinal products in preparing an SMF that meets the expectations of regulatory authorities in planning and conducting GMP inspections. The need for an SMF may vary depending on regional and national regulatory requirements, and manufacturers should consult these requirements for clarification. These guidelines apply to all types of manufacturing operations, including production, packaging and labeling, testing, relabeling, and repackaging of medicinal products. The guidelines may also be useful for blood and tissue establishments, as well as manufacturers of active pharmaceutical ingredients (APIs).

I. General Information on the Manufacturer

1. Contact information on the manufacturer
    - The manufacturer's name and official address
    - The names and street addresses of the site, buildings, and production units located on the site
    - Contact information for the manufacturer, including a 24-hour telephone number for contact personnel in the case of product defects or recalls
    - Identification numbers of the site, such as GPS details, D-U-N-S number, or any geographical location system
2. Authorized pharmaceutical manufacturing activities of the site
    - A copy of the valid manufacturing authorization issued by the relevant competent authority in Annex 1 or reference to the Eudra GMP database, if applicable. If the competent authority does not issue manufacturing authorizations, this should be stated.
    - A brief description of manufacturing, import, export, distribution, and other authorized activities by the relevant competent authorities, including foreign authorities with authorized dosage forms/activities, respectively, not covered by the manufacturing authorization.
    - The type of products currently manufactured on-site (listed in Annex 2) if not covered by Annex 1 or the Eudra GMP database.
    - A list of GMP inspections of the site within the last five years, including dates and the name/country of the competent authority that performed the inspection. A copy of the current GMP certificate should also be included.

3. Any other manufacturing activities carried out on the site
   - Description of any non-pharmaceutical activities on the site, if any.

II. Quality Management

1. The Quality Management System of the Manufacturer

Quality Management System: This section provides a brief description of the quality management systems used by the manufacturer, including references to the relevant standards. It also outlines the responsibilities of senior management for maintaining the quality system, as well as information on the site's accreditations and certifications.

2. Release Procedure of Finished Products

This section details the qualifications required for authorized persons/ qualified persons responsible for batch certification and release procedures. It also includes a general description of the batch certification and release process, the role of authorized persons/qualified persons in quarantine and release of finished products, and the arrangements in place when multiple authorized persons/qualified persons are involved. The statement also covers whether the control strategy employs process analytical technology (PAT) and/or real-time release or parametric release.

3. Management of Suppliers and Contractors

This section provides a summary of the manufacturer's supply chain and external audit program, along with a description of the qualification system for contractors, manufacturers of APIs, and other critical materials suppliers. It also outlines measures taken to ensure that products are compliant with transmitting animal spongiform encephalopathy (TSE) guidance and what happens when substandard medical products, bulk products, APIs, or excipients are suspected or identified. The use of outside scientific, analytical, or other technical assistance about manufacture and analysis is discussed, along with a list of contract manufacturers and laboratories, their addresses, and contact information. The responsibility sharing between the contract giver and acceptor is also covered, concerning compliance with the marketing authorization.

4. Quality Risk Management

This section provides a brief description of the quality risk management (QRM) methodologies used by the manufacturer, including the scope and focus of QRM, any activities performed at the corporate level, and those performed locally. It also mentions whether the QRM system has been used to assess the continuity of supply.

5. Product Quality Reviews

This section briefly describes the methodologies used for product quality reviews.

Personnel: This section includes an organization chart showing the arrangements for quality management, production, quality control positions, senior management, and authorized persons/qualified persons. It also provides the number of employees engaged in quality management, production, quality control, storage, and distribution.

6. Premises and Equipment

This section provides a short description of the plant, including the size of the site and a list of buildings. If the production takes place in different buildings for different markets, the buildings are listed with destined markets identified. It also provides a simple plan or description of manufacturing areas with an indication of scale, along with layouts and flowcharts of the production areas showing the room classification and pressure differentials between adjoining areas and indicating the production activities in the rooms. The layouts of warehouses and storage areas, with special areas for the storage and handling of highly toxic, hazardous, and sensitizing materials are indicated, if applicable. Specific storage conditions, if applicable, are also described, along with a brief description of heating, ventilation, and air-conditioning (HVAC) systems, including principles for defining the air supply, temperature, humidity, pressure differentials, and air-change rates and policy of air recirculation.

7. Details of Documentation System and Storage Location

This section requires a description of the documentation system in use, whether electronic or manual. Additionally, it should provide information on where documents and records are stored or archived off-site, including pharmacovigilance data where applicable. This should include a list of document types/records, the name and address of the storage site, and an estimate of the time required to retrieve documents from the off-site archive.

8. Production Details

This section should provide information on the type of products manufactured on-site, including a list of dosage forms of both human and veterinary products. It should also cover investigational medicinal products (IMP) manufactured for any clinical trials on the site. If different from commercial manufacturing, information on production areas and personnel should also be included. Additionally, details on toxic or hazardous substances handled, product types manufactured in a dedicated facility or on a campaign basis, and PAT applications (if applicable) should be provided. This section should also outline the general policy for process validation and the policy for reprocessing or reworking.

9. Material Management and Warehousing

This section should provide information on the arrangements for the handling of starting materials, packaging materials, bulk, and finished products. It should cover aspects such as sampling, quarantine, release, and storage. Additionally, the arrangements for the handling of rejected materials and products should be included.

10. Quality Control

This section should describe the QC activities carried out on the site in terms of physical, chemical, microbiological, and biological testing.

11. Distribution, Complaints, Product Defects, and Recalls

This section should cover details on product distribution, including the types and locations of the companies to which the products are shipped from the site. It should also describe the system used to verify that each customer/recipient is legally entitled to receive medicinal products from the manufacturer. Furthermore, a brief description of the system to ensure appropriate environmental conditions during transit, such as temperature monitoring/control, should be included. This section should also outline the arrangements for product distribution and the methods by which product traceability is maintained. Measures taken to prevent manufacturers' products from entering into the illegal supply chain should also be detailed. Lastly, a brief description of the system for handling complaints, product defects, and recalls should be included.

12. Self-inspections

This section should provide a short description of the self-inspection system with a focus on the criteria used for selecting areas to be covered during planned inspections, practical arrangements, and follow-up activities.

DRUG MASTER FILE

Introduction

A Drug Master File (DMF) is a voluntary submission to the Food and Drug Administration (FDA) that provides confidential and detailed information about facilities, processes, or articles used in the manufacturing, processing, packaging, and storing of one or more human drugs. Although it is not required by law or FDA regulation, a DMF may be submitted at the holder's discretion. The information contained in the DMF can support various applications such as Investigational New Drug Application (IND), New Drug Application (NDA), Abbreviated New Drug Application (ANDA), Export Application, or amendments and supplements to any of these. However, it is important to note that a DMF cannot substitute for an IND, NDA, ANDA, or Export Application.

The guidelines for DMF's are provided in 21 CFR 314.420 and are intended to provide DMF holders with acceptable procedures for preparing and submitting a DMF. The guidelines discuss the types of DMF's, the required information for each type, the submission format, administrative procedures governing DMF review, and the obligations of the DMF holder. The DMF's purpose is generally to allow a third party to reference material without disclosing the contents of the file. When an applicant references its material, they should refer to the information contained in their IND, NDA, or ANDA directly rather than establishing a new DMF.

TYPES OF DRUG MASTER FILE

Type I - Manufacturing site, facilities, operating procedure, and personnel

Type II - Drug substance & intermediate, material used, and drug product

Type III - Packaging material

Type IV - Excipient, flavor, essence, colorant, & material used in the preparation

Type V - FDA accepted reference information

Type I: Manufacturing Site, Facilities, Operating Procedures, and Personnel

To assist the FDA in conducting on-site inspections of manufacturing facilities outside the US, it is recommended to submit a Type I DMF. This DMF should provide a detailed description of the manufacturing site, equipment capabilities, and operational layout. Generally, a Type I DMF is not required to describe domestic facilities, unless in special cases, such as unregistered and uninspected facilities.

The description of the site should include the actual address and a map displaying its location to the nearest city. An aerial photograph and a diagram of the site may also aid in understanding the location. A diagram highlighting major production and processing areas can be beneficial in understanding the operational layout. Equipment capabilities, application, and location should also be described, but make and model details are usually unnecessary unless the equipment is new or unique. Additionally, a diagram of key organizational elements, including manufacturing, quality control, and quality assurance positions at both the manufacturing site and corporate headquarters, is helpful.

Type II: Drug substance & intermediate, material used, and drug product

A Type II DMF is typically used to provide detailed information about a specific drug intermediate, drug substance, drug product, or type of material used in their preparation.

For Drug Substance Intermediates, Drug Substances, and Material Used in Their Preparation, the submission should follow the guidelines for Submitting Supporting Documentation in Drug Applications for the Manufacture of Drug Substances and the Format and Content of the Chemistry, Manufacturing, and Controls Section of an Application.

The submission should follow the guidelines for the Format and Content of the Chemistry, Manufacturing, and Controls Section of an Application, Submitting Documentation for the Manufacture of and Controls for Drug Products, and Submitting Samples and Analytical Data for Methods Validation.

Type III: Packaging Material

For each packaging material used in the manufacturing, processing, packaging, and storing of human drugs, a Type III DMF should be submitted. The DMF should provide a detailed description of the intended use, components, composition, and release controls of the packaging material. It should also include the names of the suppliers or fabricators of the components used and the acceptance specifications. Additionally, data supporting the acceptability of the packaging material for its intended use should be provided, following the "Guideline for Submitting Documentation for Packaging for Human Drugs and Biologics."

If toxicological data on the packaging materials are not otherwise available by cross-reference to another document, it should be included under this type of DMF.

Type IV: Excipient, Colorant, Flavor, Essence, or Material Used in Their Preparation

A Type IV DMF is intended for the submission of information relating to excipients (inactive ingredients) used in the formulation of human drugs. DMF should provide a complete description of the excipient, including its composition, specifications, and controls for release.

The names of the suppliers or fabricators of the excipient and the acceptance specifications should also be given. Data supporting the acceptability of the excipient for its intended use should also be submitted as outlined in the "Guideline for Submitting Supporting Documentation in Drug Applications for the Manufacture of Drug Substances."

Toxicological data on these materials would be included under this type of DMF, if not otherwise available by cross-reference to another document. Guidelines suggested for a Type II DMF may help prepare a Type IV DMF.

Type V: FDA Accepted Reference Information

The submission of Type V DMFs for miscellaneous or duplicate information that should be included in other types of DMFs is discouraged by the FDA. If a DMF holder intends to submit information and supporting data that does not fall under Types I through IV, they must first submit a letter of intent to the Drug Master File Staff. Following this, the FDA will contact the holder to discuss the proposed submission.

Submissions of Drug Master Files

To ensure completeness and clarity of information, a DMF submission should include a transmittal letter, administrative details, and specific information as outlined in this section. All documents in the DMF should be in English, and any information in another language must be accompanied by a certified English translation. Every page of each copy of the DMF should be numbered sequentially and dated. An updated table of contents must also be provided with each submission.

A. Transmittal Letters

A.1. Original Submissions

The submission should identify as an original submission and indicate the type of DMF as classified in Section III, along with its subject. If known, the DMF should also identify the applications it is intended to support, including the name and address of each sponsor, applicant, or holder, and all relevant document numbers. The holder or authorized representative should sign the submission, and their typewritten name and title should also be provided.

A.2. Amendments

The submission should identify as an amendment and include the DMF number, type of DMF, and the subject of the amendment. A description of the purpose of submission, such as an update, revised formula, or revised process, should be included. The holder or authorized representative should sign the submission, and their typewritten name and title should also be provided.

B. Administrative Information

B.1. For Original Submissions, the following information should be provided:

(a) Name and address of the DMF holder.

(b) Name and address of corporate headquarters.

(c) Name and address of the manufacturing/processing facility.

(d) Contact information for FDA correspondence.

(e) Name and address of any agents, if applicable.

B.2. For Amendments, the following information should be included:

(a) Identification of the submission as an amendment, including the DMF number, type of DMF, and the subject of the amendment.

(b) A description of the purpose of the submission, such as an update, revised formula, or revised process.

(c) Signature of the holder or authorized representative.

(d) Typewritten name and title of the signer.

General Information and Suggestions for Preparing a DMF

1. The environmental assessment should be included in the DMF, if applicable.
2. Stability information should be provided.
3. The DMF should be assembled and delivered in an organized and easy-to-navigate format.
4. An original and duplicate copy should be submitted for all DMF submissions. The DMF holder and their agents/representatives should also retain a complete reference copy that is identical to the submissions to FDA, maintained in the same chronological order.
5. Each volume of a DMF should generally be no more than 2 inches thick, and multivolume submissions should be numbered accordingly.
6. The preferred paper size is 8-1/2 by 11 inches. However, larger individual pages may be used when necessary to present diagrams or instructions. These pages should be folded and mounted for easy review and storage.
7. Delivery to FDA

Authorization to Refer a Drug Master File

- Before the FDA can review DMF information in support of an application, the DMF holder must submit a letter of authorization to the DMF in duplicate, permitting the FDA to refer to the DMF.
- If the holder cross-references its own DMF, the authorization letter should include the information designated by items 3, 5, 6, 7, and 8 of this section. The holder does not need to send a transmittal letter with its letter of authorization.
- The letter of authorization should contain the following:
    - The date.
    - The name of the DMF holder.
    - The DMF number.
    - The names of the persons authorized to incorporate the information in the DMF by reference.
    - The specific products covered by the DMF.

- The submission dates.
- The section numbers and/or page numbers to be referenced.
- A statement of commitment that the DMF is current and that the DMF holder will comply with the statements made in it.
- The signature of the authorizing official.
- The typed name and title of the official authorizing reference to the DMF.

DRUG MASTER FILE REVIEW

A Drug Master File (DMF) is not subject to approval or disapproval. Instead, the FDA will review DMF information only when it is referenced by an IND sponsor, an applicant for an NDA, ANDA, or Export Application, or another DMF holder. Any deficiencies found in the DMF information will be communicated to the holder, who is responsible for submitting the requested information to address the deficiencies. The DMF holder must also notify affected parties of any changes or additions to the DMF and provide an annual update on the anniversary date of the original submission. Failure to update or assure the FDA annually that previously submitted material and lists remain current can cause delays in FDA review or even closure of the DMF.

Holder Obligation

The Holder Obligation mandates that any modifications or additions related to specific customers, including changes in authorization, must be submitted in duplicate and with sufficient cross-referencing to previous submissions. The cross-reference should include details such as the date, volume, section, and/or page number that is being affected by the change or addition. This requirement helps ensure that financial institutions maintain accurate and comprehensive records, which can be used to detect and prevent illegal activities such as fraud.

The following are important regulations regarding Drug Master Files (DMFs) that must be followed by holders who submit confidential information about facilities, processes, or articles used in the manufacturing, processing, packaging, and storing of one or more human drugs:

A. Notice Required for Changes to a Drug Master File:

The holder must inform every applicant or sponsor who has referenced their DMF of any significant changes made to the DMF.

B. Listing of Persons Authorized to Refer to a Drug Master File:

The DMF should have a comprehensive list of individuals who are authorized to refer to the DMF by reference. list should be updated annually and include the holder's name, DMF number, and date of the update. The updated list should identify the name or code of the information each authorized person can incorporate and provide its location by date, volume, and page number.

C. Annual Update:

The holder must provide an annual report on the original submission's anniversary date. If the DMF's subject matter remains unchanged, the holder should state that it is current. Failure to update or confirm annually with the FDA that submitted materials and lists remain current can cause delays in FDA reviews and initiate procedures for closure.

D. Appointment of an Agent:

If an agent is appointed, the holder should provide a signed letter of appointment to the DMF containing the agent's name, address, and scope of responsibility. Domestic DMF holders are not required to appoint an agent or representative.

E. Transfer of Ownership:

To transfer DMF ownership to another party, the holder should notify the FDA and authorized persons in writing. The letter should contain the name and address of the transferee, the name of their responsible official, the effective transfer date, and the transferring official's signature and title. The new holder should submit a letter of acceptance of the transfer, update the information contained in the DMF as necessary, and include any changes related to new ownership, such as plant location and methods.

Closure of Drug Master File

A holder who wishes to close a Drug Master File (DMF) should submit a request to the Drug Master File Staff, which should include the reason for the closure and a statement that the holder's obligations have been fulfilled. The FDA may also close a DMF if it does not contain an annual update of persons authorized to incorporate the information in the DMF by reference and a list of changes made since the previous annual report. The holder will be notified of the FDA's intent to close the DMF.

Practice Questions

MCQs

1. EPDB stand for
   a. Exploratory product development brief
   b. Explain the product development brief
   c. Explain the product and discover brief
   d. Explain the parcel discover a brief

2. A document is a piece of......... , ... and .... matter.
   a. Written, Printed, Electronic
   b. Placed, written, submitted
   c. Written, printed, binder
   d. Solved, printed, checked

3. Good documentation is .... Procedure.
   a. Systemic
   b. Proper
   c. Right
   d. Continuous

4. Clearly written documents prevent
   a. Errors
   b. Misunderstanding
   c. Breach of data
   d. Deletion

5. Drug product is a finished.
   a. Dosage form
   b. Prepared form
   c. Particular form
   d. Data form

6. PDP stands for
   a. Product development plan
   b. Product development paper
   c. Paper drug product
   d. Product drug plan

7. --------- record is used as a reference standard for preparing batch manufacturing record.
   a. Product development report
   b. Master formula record
   c. Batch reconciliation report
   d. All of the above

8. --------- record should be prepared for each intermediate and API/ formulation with complete information relating to manufacturing processes.
   a. Product development report
   b. Master formula record
   c. Batch reconciliation report
   d. Batch manufacturing record

9. -------- is responsible for the implementation of SOP for MFR.
   a. Head – quality assurance
   b. Head- quality control
   c. Pharmaceutical manufacturer
   d. All of the above

10. Who is primarily responsible for the issue, entering, reviewing, and control of BMR.
    a. Officer- QA
    b. Officer -QC
    c. Officer- production
    d. All of the above

11. -------- report is essential to provide a comprehensive understanding of the product and process for FDA application reviews.
    a. MFR
    b. BMR
    c. DMF
    d. PDR

12. -------- is primarily responsible for BMR attachments.
    a. Production chemist
    b. Production officer
    c. Both a and b
    d. None of the above

13. Who is secondarily responsible for BMR attachments?
    a. Production chemist
    b. Production officer
    c. Both a and b
    d. None of the above

14. % reconciliation in batch reconciliation means
    a. Quantity, of material used in manufacturing and packaging
    b. Production of material used in manufacturing and packaging
    c. Accounting of material used in manufacturing and packaging
    d. All of the above

15. -------- record is relating to all manufacturing processes for each product and batch size to be manufactured.
    a. MFR
    b. BMR
    c. SMF
    d. DMF

16. MFR should include
    a. Product detail
    b. Manufacturing processes
    c. Packaging processes
    d. All of the above

17. COA stands for
    a. Certificate of analysis
    b. Certificate of assurance
    c. Certificate of analyte
    d. Certificate of authorization

18. The basic operational and environmental conditions applied to produce safe foods are called
    a. HACCP
    b. FSSA
    c. FSSAI
    d. GMP

19. Drug master file is of ----------- types
    a. 6
    b. 7
    c. 8
    d. 5

20. DMF is prepared by
    a. Pharmaceutical manufacturer
    b. Sponsor
    c. Investigator
    d. monitor

21. DMF stands for
    a. Drug master file
    b. Drug master formula
    c. Dose master formula
    d. Dose master file

22. DMF is submitted to
    a. VENDOR
    b. SPONSOR
    c. USFDA
    d. Not submitted to any authority

23. What is a master document in the pharmaceutical industry?
    a. DMF
    b. COA
    c. SMF
    d. BMR

24. COA is given for --------- purpose.
    a. Validation of equipment
    b. Product meets its product specification
    c. Good analysis of the manufacturer
    d. Good location and premises

25. Type 3 DMF includes -----------
    a. Manufacturing site
    b. FDA accepted reference information
    c. Packaging material
    d. Excipient, colors, flavours

26. PDR Stands for Type -----------
    a. Product Development Report
    b. Product diagnosis Report
    c. Product documentation record
    d. Process Drug Record

27. BPR stands for -----------
    a. Batch Process Record
    b. Batch Primary Record
    c. Batch Packaging Record
    d. Batch Passing Record

28. BMR stands for -----------
    a. Batch Manufacturing Record
    b. Batch Master Record
    c. Batch Process Record
    d. Batch Passing Record

29. SMF Stands for -----------
    a. Site Master Formula
    b. Site Manufacture file
    c. Site Master File
    d. Substance Master file

30. Documentation in the pharmaceutical industry covers -----------
    a. Certificate of Analysis
    b. Site Manufacture file
    c. Master formula record
    d. All the above

Short Answer Questions

Q.1. Define documentation.

Q.2. Explain the basics of GDP.

Q.3. Define master formula record.

Q.4. Define the batch number.

Q.5. What is batch manufacturing record?

Long Answer Questions

Q.1. Explain EPDB for drug substance and drug product.

Q.2. Summarize in a short product development plan and product development report.

Q.3. Define batch manufacturing record and batch packing record.

Answers to MCQs

1. a	2. a	3. a	4. a
5. a	6. a	7. b	8. d
9. a	10. d	11. d	12. a
13. b	14. c	15. a	16. d
17. a	18. d	19. d	20. a
21. a	22. c	23. a	24. b
25. c	26. a	27. c	28. a
29. c	30. d		

CHAPTER 2

Dossier Preparation and Submission

A dossier is a collection of documents that contains comprehensive scientific and technical information about a pharmaceutical product, which is required to obtain regulatory approval for marketing the product. The contents of a dossier typically include administrative, quality, non-clinical, and clinical data, as well as other relevant information such as manufacturing details, stability studies, and labeling information. The format of the dossier may vary depending on the region and the regulatory authority which can be referred to as NDA in the USA, MAA in the EU, or simply Registration Dossier in other countries.

Two main formats for preparing a dossier exist ICH-CTD and ACTD. ICH-CTD is followed by ICH countries as well as low-economic or developing nations, whereas ACTD is followed by ASEAN countries. ACTD serves as a bridge between the regulatory requirements of developed and developing nations. The harmonization of both CTD and ACTD guidelines can reduce differences and variations between both guidelines. The dossier is a comprehensive scientific document that must be submitted as part of the drug approval/market authorization process. The document is used to obtain global licensing approval/market authorization for a drug by various health authorities. The regulatory affairs department is responsible for creating, processing, compiling, and dispatching the dossier, and its filling and authorization process in emerging markets may vary depending on the region.

COMMON TECHNICAL DOCUMENT

Introduction of CTD

The Common Technical Document (CTD) is a set of specifications for the application dossier required for the registration of medicines across the United States, Europe, and Japan. It was developed by the European Medicines Agency (EMA), the Food and Drug Administration (FDA), and the Ministry of Health, Labor, and Welfare (Japan) and is maintained by the International Conference on Harmonization of Technical Requirements for Registration of Pharmaceuticals for Human Use. The CTD agreement to assemble all the quality, safety, and efficacy information in a common format has revolutionized regulatory review processes.

The CTD provides a harmonized structure and format for new product applications and serves as an information package of clinical, non-clinical, manufacturing, and technical data in the same format and content for registering new drugs in all three regions. The FDA characterizes the CTD as an essential tool to facilitate simultaneous submission in three regions, exchange of regulatory information, faster availability of new medicines, and to provide a harmonized, common format/template for the submission of technical requirements to regulatory authorities that is acceptable in all three ICH regions. Ultimately, the CTD reduces the time and resources used to compile applications and eases the preparation of electronic submissions.

General Consideration

CTD (Common Technical Document) is a harmonized format for the submission of information to relevant regulatory authorities. It serves as a template for presenting data in the dossier and provides an appropriate format for the data that have been acquired. However, CTD is not a statement of data for the application of data or a guideline that indicates what studies are required. It also does not define the content of the dossier.

When preparing a CTD, it is important to ensure that the information presented is unequivocal. The style and font size used should be large enough to be easily readable, and the document should follow the ICH guidelines for document pagination and segregation as well as submission requirements and methodology for CTD. Any abbreviations used should be listed at the end of the dossier, and proper information should be given about the source of bulk drugs used for manufacturing finished formulations.

Evolution of CTD

The evolution of the Common Technical Document (CTD) can be traced back to the efforts made by the International Conference on Harmonization of Technical Requirements for Registration of Pharmaceuticals for Human Use (ICH) over the past 15-20 years. The ICH is a global initiative that brings together regulatory authorities and the pharmaceutical industry to develop harmonized guidelines and standards for the development, registration, and post-approval of pharmaceutical products.

One of the key goals of the ICH was to develop a unified format for submitting data to regulatory authorities. Before the development of the CTD, different countries had different requirements for data submission, which often resulted in redundant data generation and increased costs for the pharmaceutical industry.

The CTD was officially signed off in November 2000, at the 10th anniversary of the ICH held in San Diego, California. The CTD represents a common format for the organization and presentation of information in a regulatory submission, to facilitate the review process by regulatory authorities.

Since its inception, the CTD has undergone several revisions and updates, including the addition of new sections and the clarification of existing guidelines. The CTD is now widely accepted and used as the standard format for the submission of data to regulatory authorities in many countries worldwide.

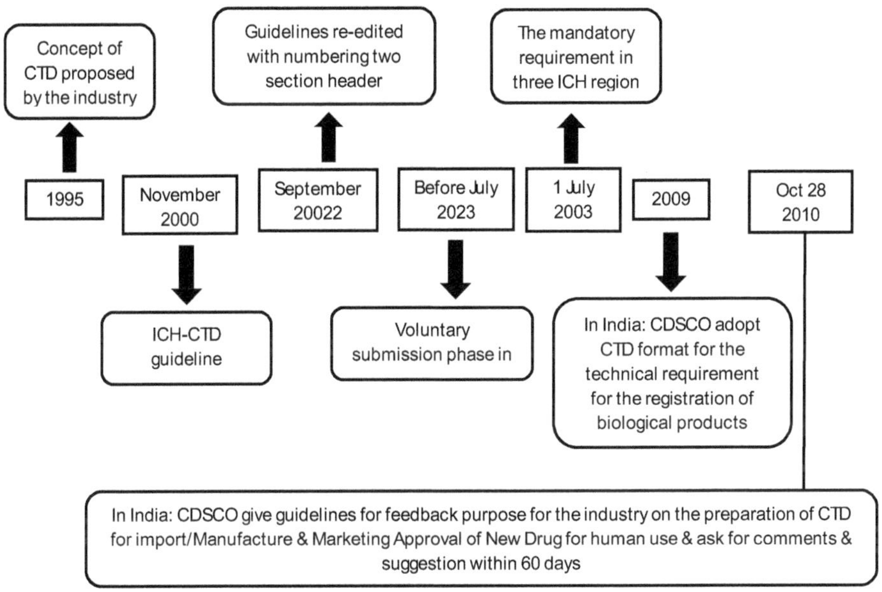

Figure 2.1 Evolution of CTD.

OVERVIEW AND MODULES OF CTD

CTD MODULES

The Common Technical Document (CTD) is organized into five modules, with Module 1 being region-specific, and Modules 2, 3, 4, and 5 being common for all regions. These modules are presented in a standard format that is acceptable to regulatory authorities in different regions.

Module 1 contains administrative information that is specific to the region in which the product is being submitted for registration. This module typically includes information such as the product name, application type, and regulatory requirements specific to the region.

Module 2 contains the Quality Overall Summary (QOS), which is a comprehensive summary of the pharmaceutical product's quality data. This module also includes information on the drug substance, drug product, and manufacturing process, among other things.

Module 3 contains information on the quality of the product, including Chemistry, Manufacturing, and Controls (CMC) data. This module includes information on the drug substance, drug product, and analytical methods used to assess product quality.

Module 4 contains non-clinical study reports, including information on the product's pharmacology, toxicology, and pharmacokinetics.

Module 5 contains clinical study reports, including information on the product's clinical efficacy, safety, and pharmacokinetics.

The modular structure of the CTD is often represented as a triangle, with Module 1 at the top of the triangle, and Modules 2-5 forming the sides of the triangle. This modular structure makes it easier for regulatory authorities to review the information provided in submission and compare products from different manufacturers.

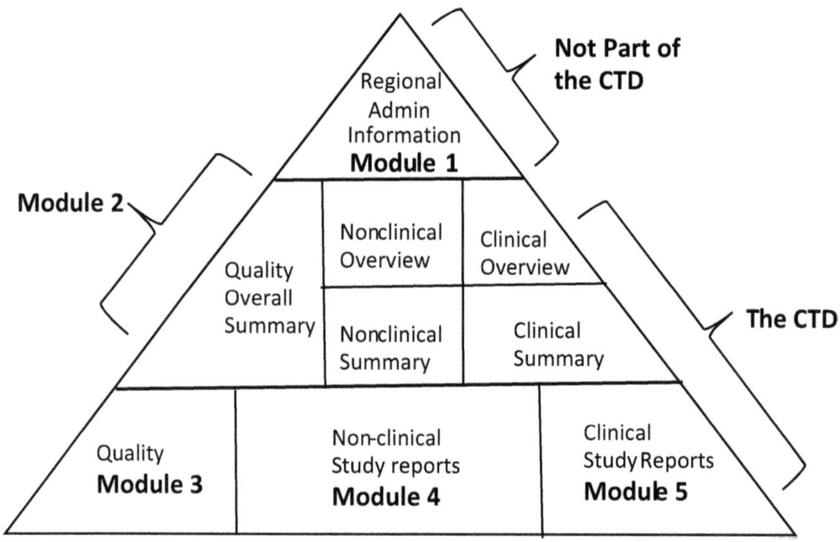

Figure 2.2 Organizational Structure of CTD.

MODULE 1: Administrative information (region-specific)

Module 1 of the Common Technical Document (CTD) contains administrative information that is specific to the region in which the pharmaceutical product is being submitted for registration. This module typically includes information such as:

1.1 Table of Contents:

This section provides a list of all the sections and subsections included in the CTD.

1.2 Body of Data:

This section provides information on the quality, safety, and efficacy of the product. It includes information on the drug substance, drug product, manufacturing process, and analytical methods used to assess product quality.

1.3 Introduction and Overall Table of Contents:

This section provides an overview of the contents of the CTD and describes the purpose of each module.

1.4 Regional Administrative Information:

This section provides information on the specific regulatory requirements for the region in which the product is being submitted. It includes information on the submission process, timelines, and any specific documentation requirements.

1.5 Product-Specific Information:

This section provides information on the specific product being submitted for registration, including the product name, dosage form, and strength.

1.6 Module 1 - Regional Information:

This section provides specific regional information, such as the product's proposed labeling, product literature, and any other regional-specific documentation.

1.7 Environmental Risk Assessment:

This section provides information on the potential environmental impact of the product, including its impact on the environment during manufacturing, distribution, and use.

Overall, Module 1 provides essential information on the administrative aspects of the submission process, including specific regional requirements, and is crucial in ensuring the successful submission and review of the CTD.

MODULE 2 CTD: Quality overall summary (QOS)

Module 2 of the Common Technical Document (CTD) is called the Quality Overall Summary (QOS). It provides a comprehensive summary of the pharmaceutical product's quality data, including information on the drug substance, drug product, and manufacturing process, among other things.

The QOS serves as a high-level overview of the product and provides a framework for the reviewer to understand the quality and safety of the product.

The QOS should be written clearly and concisely and should summarize the information contained in the other modules of the CTD.

The following are the main sections included in Module 2:

2.1 Administrative Information:

This section provides administrative information on the submission, including the product name, application type, and regulatory authority to which the submission is being made.

2.2 Table of Contents:

This section provides a list of all the sections and subsections included in the QOS.

2.3 Introduction:

This section provides an overview of the product and describes the purpose and scope of the QOS.

2.4 Quality Overall Summary:

This section summarizes the quality data for the product, including information on the drug substance, drug product, and manufacturing process. It should provide an overview of the product's quality and safety, including any critical quality attributes (CQAs) and how they are controlled.

2.5 Clinical Overview:

This section provides an overview of the product's clinical development program, including the objectives of each study, the patient population studied, and the results of the studies.

2.6 Nonclinical Overview:

This section provides an overview of the nonclinical studies conducted for the product, including information on pharmacology, toxicology, and pharmacokinetics.

2.7 Overall Conclusion:

This section provides an overall conclusion on the product's quality, safety, and efficacy based on the information provided in the QOS.

Overall, Module 2 is critical in providing an overview of the product's quality data, and it serves as a starting point for the regulatory authority's review of the submission.

MODULE 3: Quality (CMC)

Module 3 of the Common Technical Document (CTD) is dedicated to the Quality section, also known as Module 3 Quality (M3Q). It provides a harmonized structure and format for presenting chemistry, manufacturing, and controls (CMC) information in a drug product registration dossier.

The purpose of Module 3 Quality is to provide detailed information about the drug substance and drug product, including their characterization, manufacturing process, and controls. The section is divided into several sub-sections, including:

1. ***Drug Substance*:** This section describes the chemical and physical characteristics of the drug substance, including its identity, impurities, and reference standards.
2. ***Drug Product*:** This section describes the drug product formulation and manufacturing process, including the materials used, manufacturing steps, and controls.
3. ***Container Closure System*:** This section describes the primary packaging materials used for the drug product and their compatibility with the drug substance and drug product.
4. ***Manufacturing*:** This section provides detailed information on the manufacturing process, including process controls, validation data, and a description of the manufacturing facility.
5. ***Control of Materials*:** This section describes the controls used to ensure the quality and purity of the raw materials used in the manufacturing process.
6. ***Control of Critical Steps and Intermediates*:** This section describes the controls used to ensure the quality and consistency of critical manufacturing steps and intermediates.
7. ***Control of Drug Product*:** This section describes the controls used to ensure the quality and consistency of the final drug product, including the analytical methods used to test the product and the acceptance criteria.
8. ***Stability and Shelf Life*:** This section provides data on the stability of the drug product, including stability protocol, storage conditions, and results of stability testing.

Overall, Module 3 Quality is a critical component of the CTD and provides a comprehensive description of the drug substance and drug product, manufacturing process, and controls. It helps regulatory authorities evaluate the quality, safety, and efficacy of the drug product and ensures a harmonized approach to the presentation of CMC information in a registration dossier.

MODULE 4 Non-Clinical Study Reports.

Module 4 of the Common Technical Document (CTD) is dedicated to Nonclinical Study Reports, also known as Module 4 (M4). The purpose of Module 4 is to provide a detailed summary of the nonclinical studies performed with the drug substance and drug product, including pharmacology, toxicology, and pharmacokinetic studies.

The Nonclinical Study Reports section is divided into several sub-sections, including:

1. ***Introduction***: This section provides an overview of the nonclinical studies performed and their relevance to human safety and efficacy.
2. ***Pharmacology***: This section provides data on the pharmacological properties of the drug substance and drug product, including their mechanism of action, pharmacodynamics, and pharmacokinetics.
3. ***Toxicology***: This section provides data on the toxicological properties of the drug substance and drug product, including acute, sub-chronic, and chronic toxicity, as well as genotoxicity, carcinogenicity, and reproductive toxicity.
4. ***Safety Pharmacology***: This section provides data on the effects of the drug substance and drug product on vital organ systems, such as the cardiovascular, respiratory, and central nervous systems.
5. ***Pharmacokinetics***: This section provides data on the absorption, distribution, metabolism, and excretion of the drug substance and drug product in animal models.
6. ***Local Tolerance***: This section provides data on the local tissue reactions of the drug substance and drug product, including irritation, sensitization, and local toxicity.
7. ***Other Studies***: This section provides data on any additional nonclinical studies performed, such as immunotoxicity or pharmacogenomics.

Overall, Module 4 provides a comprehensive overview of the nonclinical studies performed with the drug substance and drug product, which helps regulatory authorities evaluate the safety and efficacy of the drug product before human testing is initiated.

MODULE 5: Clinical Study Reports

Module 5 of the Common Technical Document (CTD) is dedicated to Clinical Study Reports (CSR), also known as Module 5 (M5). The purpose of Module 5 is to provide a detailed summary of the clinical studies performed with the drug product, including safety and efficacy data, in support of the marketing application.

The Clinical Study Reports section is divided into several sub-sections, including:

1. ***Introduction***: This section provides an overview of the clinical studies performed and their relevance to human safety and efficacy.
2. ***Study Reports***: This section provides detailed reports on each of the clinical studies performed, including study design, patient characteristics, efficacy and safety results, adverse events, and statistical analyses.

3. ***Integrated Summary of Efficacy*:** This section provides a summary of the efficacy data from all clinical studies performed, including pooled analyses and subgroup analyses.
4. ***Integrated Summary of Safety*:** This section provides a summary of the safety data from all clinical studies performed, including adverse events, serious adverse events, and laboratory abnormalities.
5. ***Clinical Overview*:** This section provides an integrated summary of the clinical data, including efficacy, safety, and risk-benefit analysis, and discusses the clinical implications of the data.

Overall, Module 5 provides a comprehensive overview of the clinical studies performed with the drug product, which helps regulatory authorities evaluate the safety and efficacy of the drug product and its potential risks and benefits to patients.

Electronic Dossier Submission Process and Validating the Submission

The electronic dossier submission process involves submitting the CTD electronically to regulatory authorities using the Electronic Common Technical Document (eCTD) format. The eCTD is a standardized format that allows for easy and efficient electronic submission of the CTD.

To submit the eCTD, the following steps are typically involved:

1. ***Convert the CTD into eCTD format*:** The CTD is converted into eCTD format using software tools such as eCTD submission software.
2. ***Validate the eCTD*:** The eCTD is validated to ensure that it meets the regulatory authority's technical requirements for submission. The validation process checks for errors, inconsistencies, and formatting issues in the eCTD.
3. ***Submit the eCTD*:** Once the eCTD has been validated and any errors corrected, it is submitted electronically to the regulatory authority.
4. ***Tracking the submission*:** It is important to keep track of the submission and ensure that it has been received by the regulatory authority. Most regulatory authorities provide an electronic tracking system to monitor the status of the submission.

The validation process is critical to ensure the quality and accuracy of the eCTD submission. The validation process involves several steps, including:

1. ***Technical validation*:** This step checks the technical requirements of the eCTD, including file names, file types, and file sizes.
2. ***Format validation*:** This step checks the format and structure of the eCTD to ensure that it complies with the regulatory authority's specifications.
3. ***Content validation*:** This step checks the content of the eCTD to ensure that it includes all the required information and that the information is accurate and consistent.

4. ***Business rule validation***: This step checks the eCTD against the business rules of the regulatory authority to ensure that it complies with their specific requirements

Overall, the eCTD submission process and validation process are critical to ensure the timely and efficient review of the CTD by regulatory authorities.

ELECTRONIC COMMON TECHNICAL DOCUMENT

The Electronic Common Technical Document (eCTD) is a standardized format for the electronic submission of regulatory information to health authorities. The eCTD was developed by the International Conference on Harmonization (ICH) and is used by regulatory authorities worldwide.

The eCTD is a structured format that organizes regulatory information into electronic folders, which are based on the CTD. It allows for the efficient electronic submission of regulatory information and simplifies the review process for regulatory authorities.

The eCTD consists of a set of XML files and associated documents, which are organized into five main sections, or modules, that correspond to the CTD modules:

1. ***Module 1 - Administrative information***: This module contains administrative and procedural information about the submission, such as cover letters, application forms, and authorization letters.
2. ***Module 2 - Summaries***: This module contains summaries of the information presented in the other modules, such as the quality, non-clinical, and clinical information.
3. ***Module 3 - Quality***: This module contains information about the quality of the drug substance and drug product, such as manufacturing and control information.
4. ***Module 4 - Non-clinical study reports***: This module contains information about non-clinical studies conducted on the drug substance and drug product.
5. ***Module 5 - Clinical study reports***: This module contains information about clinical studies conducted on the drug substance and drug product

The eCTD format allows for the efficient review and processing of regulatory submissions by regulatory authorities. It also facilitates the sharing of information between regulatory authorities and enables the use of electronic tools for document management and review.

Overall, the eCTD is an important tool for the electronic submission of regulatory information and plays a critical role in the drug development and regulatory approval process.

CTD → TOC (pdf) (paper)

eCTD → XML Backbone

The eCTD format is a standardized electronic format for submitting regulatory information related to drug products. It follows the Common Technical Document (CTD) format and was developed by the International Conference on Harmonization (ICH) M2 Expert Working Group. The eCTD format is widely used for submitting applications, amendments, supplements, and reports to regulatory agencies such as the US FDA and the European Medicines Agency (EMA). The use of eCTD is mandatory for many types of submissions in the US, and it is also required for all procedures in the European Union since 2010.

CTD		e CTD
MODULE 1		m1
MODULE 2	→	m2
MODULE 3	→	m3
MODULE 4	→	m4
MODULE 5		m5

eCTD Characteristics

Structure

The eCTD format offers several characteristics that make it an effective way to submit regulatory information related to drug products. One of these is the structure of the format. All modules of the CTD (Modules 1 to 5) have granularity options, which allow for greater flexibility in presenting information.

Another characteristic of eCTD is that it allows for the use of PDF documents linked via an XML backbone. This means that the submission is transparent and easy to navigate and review, and the entire submission can be accessed and viewed electronically. Additionally, the increased document granularity in eCTD allows for more precise targeting of specific sections of the submission, which can save time and resources during the review process.

Benefits of eCTD

- Increased efficiency in the review process by regulatory authorities.
- Reduced paper-based submission and storage requirements.
- Improved data quality and accuracy through the use of standardized formats.

- Faster time to market for pharmaceutical products due to streamlined submission process.
- Improved consistency and completeness of regulatory submissions.
- Improved global collaboration and harmonization in regulatory processes.
- Easier tracking and monitoring of regulatory submissions and status updates.
- Improved security and confidentiality of submitted data.

Document Granularity- Module 1

Module 1 of an eCTD submission is a crucial part of the dossier that contains administrative and prescribing information related to the drug. It serves as an index to the entire submission and provides essential details that regulatory agencies use to track the application. The following are the key components of Module 1:

1. ***Application form*:** This section includes the company's name, the drug name, the submission type, the date of application, and the sequence number assigned by the regulatory agency.
2. ***Regional administrative information*:** This section contains administrative details specific to the region where the submission is made, such as the product license number and the date of approval.
3. ***Product information*:** This section includes the drug's formulation, strength, route of administration, and dosage form.
4. ***Prescribing information*:** This section provides information on how to use the drug, including the indications, dosage, administration, warnings, precautions, and contraindications.
5. ***Quality information*:** This section contains information on the drug's manufacturing process, stability data, and analytical methods used for quality control.
6. ***Nonclinical study reports*:** This section includes nonclinical study reports and summaries of toxicology and pharmacology studies.
7. ***Clinical study reports*:** This section includes clinical study reports and summaries of the drug's clinical trials, including data on safety, efficacy, and pharmacokinetics.
8. ***Appendices*:** This section contains supporting documents, such as product labels, certificates of analysis, and reference publications.

The granularity of the document in Module 1 should be at a high level to ensure that all necessary information is included while avoiding unnecessary duplication or inclusion of extraneous data. The information in Module 1 should be concise and easily accessible to regulatory agencies to facilitate the review process.

Summaries- Module 2

Module 2 in eCTD format contains the summaries of the drug development process. It is divided into five sections, as follows:

1. ***Clinical Summaries*:** This section includes a summary of clinical trials conducted during the drug development process. It includes information about the trial design, study population, efficacy, and safety data, along with any statistical analyses conducted.
2. ***Nonclinical Summaries*:** This section includes a summary of nonclinical studies conducted during the drug development process. It includes information about the pharmacology, toxicology, and other nonclinical data, along with any statistical analyses conducted.
3. ***Quality Overall Summary (QOS)*:** This section includes a summary of the drug product's quality, manufacturing, and controls. It includes information about the drug substance, drug product, analytical methods, and manufacturing process, as well as any stability data.
4. ***Analytical Summaries*:** This section includes a summary of the analytical methods used to test the drug substance and drug product. It includes information about the methods used, their validation, and any results obtained.
5. ***Clinical Overview*:** This section provides an overview of the clinical development program for the drug. It includes a summary of the key clinical data, the clinical safety and efficacy profile, and any unresolved issues or questions related to the clinical development program.

Module 2 is an important part of the eCTD submission, as it provides a comprehensive summary of the drug development process and the data that support the safety and efficacy of the drug product. The information in Module 2 is used by regulatory authorities to assess the safety and efficacy of the drug and to make a decision about whether to approve the drug for marketing.

Document Granularity - Module 3

Module 3 in eCTD is focused on providing detailed information about the quality, nonclinical, and clinical aspects of the drug product being submitted. This module is a crucial part of any eCTD submission as it contains information on the safety, efficacy, and quality of the drug product.

The documents included in Module 3 may vary depending on the type of drug being submitted and the specific regulatory requirements of the region where the submission is being made. However, some common types of documents that may be included in Module 3 are:

1. ***Quality Documents*:** This section contains all the information related to the quality of the drug product. This includes drug substance and drug product manufacturing, testing and control, stability data, impurities, and specifications.

2. ***Nonclinical Study Reports*:** This section contains reports of all nonclinical studies conducted on the drug product. This includes pharmacology, toxicology, pharmacokinetics, and metabolism studies.
3. ***Clinical Study Reports*:** This section contains reports of all clinical trials conducted on the drug product. This includes the protocol, investigator brochure, clinical study reports, and statistical analysis.
4. ***Clinical Summaries*:** This section contains summary documents that provide a concise overview of the clinical data. This includes clinical study reports, clinical overview, clinical summary, and integrated summary of safety and efficacy.
5. ***Other Documents*:** Other documents that may be included in Module 3 are environmental risk assessment reports, pediatric study plans, and risk management plans.

In summary, Module 3 of eCTD is focused on providing detailed information about the safety, efficacy, and quality of the drug product being submitted. It contains a variety of documents that provide information on nonclinical and clinical studies, quality data, and other relevant information necessary for the regulatory evaluation of the drug product.

Document Granularity - Modules 4

Module 4 of an eCTD submission contains the nonclinical study reports. This module includes data from animal studies, such as pharmacology, toxicology, and pharmacokinetics. It also includes information on the formulation of the drug product, the manufacturing process, and stability data. Module 4 is divided into several sections, including:

1. ***Nonclinical Overview*:** This section provides an overall summary of the nonclinical studies conducted on the drug product.
2. ***Pharmacology Studies*:** This section contains information on the drug's mechanism of action, its pharmacodynamic and pharmacokinetic properties, and its effects on various physiological systems.
3. ***Toxicology Studies*:** This section contains data from toxicology studies conducted on animals to evaluate the safety of the drug. It includes information on acute toxicity, repeated dose toxicity, carcinogenicity, and reproductive and developmental toxicity.
4. ***Pharmacokinetics Studies*:** This section contains data on the drug's absorption, distribution, metabolism, and excretion in animals.
5. ***Safety Pharmacology Studies*:** This section contains data from studies conducted to evaluate the drug's effects on various physiological systems, such as cardiovascular, respiratory, and central nervous systems.
6. ***Ecotoxicity and Environmental Risk Assessment*:** This section contains data on the potential impact of the drug on the environment, including its effects on aquatic organisms and the environment in general.

7. ***Environmental Risk Assessment***: This section contains an assessment of the potential environmental risks associated with the use of the drug product.

Overall, Module 4 provides a comprehensive overview of the nonclinical data that supports the safety and efficacy of the drug product.

Contains Clinical Study Data - Module 5

Module 5 of the eCTD format contains clinical study reports and data from clinical trials conducted for the drug. This module is further divided into several sections, including:

1. ***Study Reports***: This section contains the full reports for each clinical study conducted, including study protocols, statistical analysis plans, and final study reports.
2. ***Investigator's Brochures***: This section contains the investigator's brochure, which is a comprehensive document providing information about the drug, its development, pharmacological and toxicological effects, and clinical trials conducted.
3. ***Clinical Summaries***: This section contains summaries of the clinical studies conducted for the drug, including clinical trial reports, integrated summaries of safety and efficacy, and clinical overviews.
4. ***Nonclinical Study Reports***: This section contains reports of the nonclinical studies conducted for the drug, including toxicology and pharmacology studies.

Overall, Module 5 provides critical information about the safety and efficacy of the drug, which is crucial for regulatory authorities to assess before approving the drug for marketing.

Module 5 contains a comprehensive collection of clinical study data, which is submitted to regulatory agencies to demonstrate the safety and efficacy of a drug. This module is typically submitted as part of a marketing authorization application (MAA) or a new drug application (NDA). The documents in Module 5 are presented in a granular format to provide an in-depth understanding of the clinical trial data.

The key documents in Module 5 include clinical study reports, which provide a detailed description of the study design, methods, and results. The clinical study report is presented in a standard format, including a synopsis, study report, and other annexes.

Other documents in Module 5 include the protocol and amendment, sample case report form, list of IECs or IRBs, and consent form. There is also a listing of investigation sites, patient data, statistical methods, and audit certificates. Publications based on the study, important references, discontinued patients, protocol deviations, and demographic data are also included.

Additionally, Module 5 contains compliance and drug concentration data, individual efficacy response data, and adverse event listings. There is also a listing of individual laboratory measurements by patient. All of these documents provide a detailed and comprehensive overview of the clinical study data, which is essential for regulatory agencies to evaluate the safety and efficacy of a drug.

Document Publishing

PDF files created from intelligent sources such as MS Office should be text searchable. However, some legacy documents may only be available in scanned form, which means they are essentially images of the original document and not text searchable. In this case, the file name should be compared with the document contents to ensure accuracy. It is important to ensure that all documents are in the appropriate format and are properly labeled and organized in the eCTD submission to ensure efficient review and approval by regulatory authorities.

In PDF Check Page Size and Orientation

The page size and orientation in the PDF files should match the paper size and orientation of the original documents. However, in the case of electronic submissions, the US FDA accepts A4-sized PDF documents in eCTD submissions, even though the standard paper size in the US is letter-sized. On the other hand, the EU member states require A4 paper dossiers, but they accept letter-sized PDFs in eCTD submissions. It's important to check the requirements of the regulatory agency where the submission will be made to ensure compliance.

Submitting the eCTD

To submit an eCTD, you need to include a cover letter (in PDF format) based on the ICH eCTD specification version 3.2.2. The cover letter should also be provided as a paper copy, along with any non-electronic parts of the submission. In addition to the cover letter, you should describe the submission that includes relevant regulatory information. You should also indicate which sections of the submission are filed as paper, electronic, or both. Furthermore, you need to describe the electronic submission in terms of the type and number of electronic media used, the approximate size of the submission, and any relevant characteristics of the media (such as the format used for DLT tapes), based on regional guidance. You should also state that the submission is virus-free and describe the software used to check the files for viruses. Finally, you need to provide the regulatory and information technology points of contact for the submission. To create eCTD copies, you should copy the eCTD to a CD-ROM, DVD, or DLT master, reload it from the master, and revalidate it. The number of copies required by each EU member state may vary.

When submitting an eCTD, you should prepare a cover letter in both paper and PDF formats, based on the ICH eCTD specification version 3.2.2. The cover letter should be accompanied by any non-electronic parts of the submission and should describe the submission that includes relevant regulatory information. You should also indicate which parts of the submission are electronic, paper, or both, and provide details about the electronic media used, including the type, number, size, and format (if applicable) of the media. Make sure to state that the submission is free of viruses and provide information about the virus-checking software used. You should also include the regulatory and information technology points of contact for the submission. To create eCTD copies, you should copy the submission to a CD-ROM, DVD, or DLT master, reload it from the master, and revalidate it. The number of copies required may vary depending on the requirements of each EU member state.

Submitting an eCTD involves several steps. First, you need to prepare a cover letter that complies with the ICH eCTD specification version 3.2.2. The cover letter should be provided in both paper and PDF formats, along with any non-electronic parts of the submission. In the cover letter, you should describe the submission and provide relevant regulatory information. You should also indicate which parts of the submission are electronic, paper, or both. Additionally, you need to provide details about the electronic media used, including the type, number, size, and format (if applicable) of the media, based on regional guidance. It's important to ensure that the submission is virus-free and to describe the virus-checking software used. Finally, you should include the regulatory and information technology points of contact for the submission. Once you have prepared the submission, you should copy the eCTD to a CD-ROM, DVD, or DLT master, reload it from the master, and revalidate it. Depending on the requirements of each EU member state, you may need to create multiple copies of the eCTD.

Points to Remember

1. Make sure to include all files referenced in the XML backbone(s) in the eCTD submission.
2. Module 1 is mandatory in all eCTD submissions and should include a company name, drug name, submission type, date of application, and sequence number.
3. Application numbers must be 6 digits long.
4. Sequence numbers must be 4 digits long.
5. Verify that the submission received by the regulatory authority matches the intended submission.
6. Do not submit a single eCTD for multiple applications.
7. XML components must conform to standard specifications.

8. PDF documents should have recognizable text.
9. Check that all hyperlinks and bookmarks in PDF documents are accurate.
10. PDF documents should have a table of contents.

FILE FORMATS SHOULD USE FOR ELECTRONIC DOCUMENTS

1. PDF Version

   All PDF files should be readable with version 3.0 of the Acrobat Reader, with the search plug-in. Additional software should not be required to read and navigate the PDF file.

2. Font Usage

   To limit storage space taken by embedded fonts, consider the following:

   - Limit the number of fonts used in each document
   - Use only True Type or Adobe Type 1 font
   - Avoid customized fonts
   - Use black font color. The blue font may be used for hypertext links (preferred for submissions to CBER).
   - If a font color other than black is used, avoid light colors that do not print well on grayscale printers.

3. Orientation

   Ensure all documents are correctly oriented for on-screen display and all pages in an individual document have the same orientation. Clearly and uniquely label all documents and drawings and include version/issue numbers (e.g., title, drawing number, and version/issue) in separate, clearly labeled files.

4. Page Size and Margins

   The print area for pages should fit on a sheet of paper that is 8.5 inches by 11 inches. Maintain a margin of at least 1 inch on all sides to avoid obscuring information if the pages are subsequently printed and bound.

5. Source of Electronic Document

   PDF documents produced from an electronic source document are superior to those produced by scanning paper documents. Scanned documents are difficult to read and do not allow us to search or copy and paste text for editing. They should be avoided if at all possible.

6. Methods for Creating

   PDF Documents and Images Choose a method for creating PDF documents that produce the best replication of a paper document. Ensure that the paper and PDF versions of the document are the same by printing the document from the PDF version. When creating PDF files containing images, do not resample images.

7. Hypertext Linking and Bookmarks

   Hypertext links and bookmarks are techniques used to improve navigation through PDF documents. Hypertext links can be designated by rectangles using thin lines or by blue text. When creating bookmarks and hyperlinks, choose the magnification setting Inherit Zoom so that the destination page displays at the same magnification level that the reviewer is using for the rest of the document.

8. Page Numbering

   If a submission includes more than one document, provide page numbers only for individual documents.

9. Document Information Fields

   Use document information fields to search for individual documents and to identify the document when found.

10. Naming PDF Files

    Use recommended names to avoid misunderstandings, improve communication, and speed up the review of a submission. If the file name is not specified, use names up to 32 characters in length with a 3-character extension. Avoid using punctuation, spaces, or other nonalphanumeric symbols in file names.

11. Security

    Do not include any security settings or password protection for PDF files. Allow printing, changes to the document, selecting text and graphics, and adding or changing notes and form fields. Internal security and archival processes will maintain the integrity of the submitted files.

12. Indexing PDF Documents

    Use full-text indexes to help find specific documents and/or search for text within documents. When a document or group of documents is indexed, all words and numbers in the file and all information stored in the Document Information fields are stored in special index files that are functionally accessible using the search tools available in Acrobat.

13. Electronic Signatures

    We are developing procedures for archiving documents with electronic signatures. Until those procedures are in place, documents requiring an original signature, such as certifications, must be accompanied by a paper copy that includes the handwritten signature and the submission identifier (e.g., NDA number).

VALIDATION

Validation is a process by which the FDA performs checks to ensure that electronic submissions are accurate and processed correctly. These checks apply to both eCTD and non-eCTD submissions and include verifying that the application form matches the specified application type in the us-regional.xml file. For example, if the us-regional.xml specifies an NDA application type, but the sponsor submits a form 1571, additional validation checks will be performed. Additionally, the FDA ensures that the application number specified in the us-regional.xml file is consistent with the application form. These checks are performed to ensure that submissions are processed and routed accurately and in a timely fashion.

ASEAN COMMON TECHNICAL DOCUMENT [ACTD]

Introduction

The ASEAN Common Technical Document (ACTD) is a set of guidelines established by the Association of Southeast Asian Nations (ASEAN) for the registration of pharmaceuticals in the ASEAN region. The ACTD is designed to provide a harmonized format for the preparation of regulatory submissions, making it easier for pharmaceutical companies to register their products across multiple ASEAN countries.

The ASEAN Common Technical Document (ACTD) is a standardized format and structure for compiling the documentation required for a marketing authorization application in the ASEAN region. Its purpose is to provide a common format and structure that can be used by applicants to submit their dossiers consistently and efficiently. The ACTD guides the organization and content of the dossier but does not provide recommendations on the actual content of the documents included in the dossier.

The ACTD is similar to the European Union's Common Technical Document (EU-CTD) and is intended to simplify the regulatory process by providing a consistent format across all ASEAN member countries. The ACTR, or ASEAN Common Technical Requirements, is a set of guidelines intended to help applicants prepare their dossiers by the expectations of all ASEAN drug regulatory authorities. It guides the content and quality of the data and information required for a successful application.

The ACTD consists of five modules, each of which contains information on specific aspects of the pharmaceutical registration process. These modules include:

1. ***Module 1 - Administrative Information*:** This module includes information such as the application form, product information, and labeling information.
2. ***Module 2 - Quality overall summary*:** This module provides an overview of the quality control and quality assurance aspects of the pharmaceutical product.

3. ***Module 3 - Nonclinical study reports*:** This module includes information on the nonclinical studies conducted on the product, such as toxicology studies and pharmacokinetic studies.
4. ***Module 4 - Clinical study reports*:** This module includes information on the clinical studies conducted on the product, such as clinical trial protocols, study results, and adverse events.
5. ***Module 5 - Common technical document summaries*:** This module includes a summary of the information contained in Modules 2, 3, and 4, as well as any additional information required by the regulatory authorities in each ASEAN country.

By following the ACTD guidelines, pharmaceutical companies can streamline the regulatory submission process, reducing the time and cost involved in registering products in the ASEAN region.

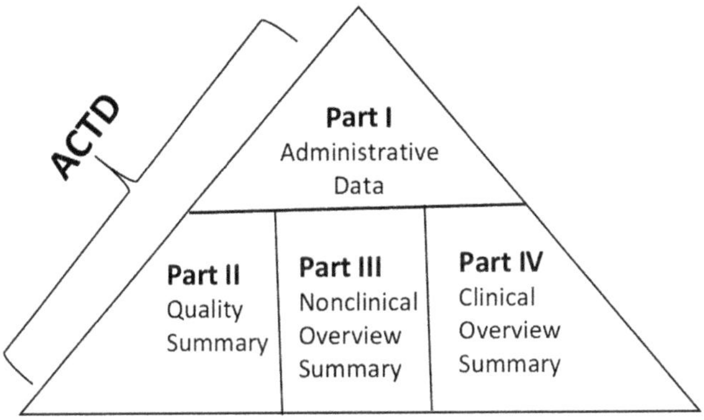

Figure 2.3 Organizational Structure of ACTD.

Practice Questions

MCQs

1. CTD stands for
   a. Central technical document
   b. Common technical document
   c. Centre technical document
   d. Common technical dossier
2. The CTD is organized into..........modules.
   a. 4
   b. 2
   c. 5
   d. 3

3. Module 1 contains
   a. CTD Summaries (QOS)
   b. Administration information (region-specific)
   c. Quality
   d. clinical study Reports

4. Module 2 contain
   a. CTD Summaries
   b. Nonclinical Study Reports
   c. Quality
   d. Administration information

5. Module 5 contain
   a. CTD Summaries
   b. clinical study Reports
   c. Nonclinical Study Reports
   d. Administration information

6. eCTD stand for
   a. electronic common technical document
   b. electronic central technical document
   c. electronic common technical dossier
   d. electro common technical document

7. eCTD composed of.......... types of specification.
   a. 1
   b. 5
   c. 2
   d. 4

8. Submission in eCTD format should be by the current ICH M2 EWG eCTD specification.
   a. True
   b. False

9. CTD is highly recommended by USFDA for NDAs, BLAs, DMFs, and INDs filing.
   a. True
   b. False

10. The eCTD is organized into...........modules.
    a. 1
    b. 2
    c. 5
    d. 3

11. Benefits of eCTD
    a. Easy to distribute and review.
    b. More efficient use of resources, less cost, and stress to the organization.
    c. Highly organized electronic tablet of contents.
    d. All of the above

12. The word 'Dossier' has the English meaning as a collection or file of documents on a particular subject, especially a file containing detailed information about a person or a topic.

    a. True   b. False

13. The CTD is maintained by the International Conference on Harmonization of Technical Requirements for Registration of Pharmaceuticals for Human Use.

    a. True   b. False

Short Answer Questions

Q.1. Short note on CTD and ACTD modules.

Q.2. Define Electronic gateway (ECG).

Q.3. Short note on Electronic dossier submission.

Q.4. Explain Submission in the sugar system of CDSCO.

Long Answer Questions

Q1. Explain in detail the modules of CTD and eCTD.

Q.2 Identify the steps involved in electronic submission gateway (ESG) and Asian CTD formats submission.

Answers to MCQs

1. d	2. c	3. b	4. a
5. b	6. a	7. c	8. a
9. a	10. c	11. d	12. a
13. a			

CHAPTER 3

Audits

An audit is essentially an examination of a company's financial or operational records to ensure that they are accurate and comply with relevant laws and regulations. However, audits can also be conducted in other areas, such as quality management, environmental management, and information security, among others. The purpose of an audit is to provide an independent and objective assessment of a company's processes, controls, and systems to identify areas for improvement and ensure compliance with applicable standards or regulations.

Audits are systematic and objective evaluations of a process, system, organization, or product to determine the extent to which they comply with established criteria or standards. The purpose of an audit is to identify areas of improvement, evaluate the effectiveness of controls and ensure compliance with regulations, policies, or standards. Audits can be conducted internally by an organization's personnel or by external third-party auditors. Some common types of audits include financial audits, operational audits, compliance audits, and quality audits. Audits may be conducted regularly or in response to specific incidents or concerns. The results of an audit are typically documented in an audit report, which outlines any findings, recommendations, or corrective actions needed to address identified issues.

QUALITY AUDIT

Quality audits are an essential part of quality management systems and are conducted to assess the effectiveness of the system, identify areas for improvement, and ensure compliance with relevant standards, regulations, and guidelines. The focus of quality audits is on the processes and systems that produce the product or service rather than the product or service itself. The goal is to ensure that the quality system is working as intended and that the organization is meeting its quality objectives.

A quality audit is a process that examines and evaluates an organization's quality management system to determine whether it is meeting established quality standards and regulations. It is a systematic and independent examination of the organization's quality management system, procedures, and processes to ensure they are effective, efficient, and in compliance with the relevant regulatory requirements and standards. The purpose of a quality audit is to identify areas of improvement in the quality system and to ensure that the organization is meeting its quality objectives. Quality audits can be conducted internally by an organization's quality assurance team or externally by a third-party auditor.

Audit Policy

An audit policy is a set of guidelines and procedures designed to ensure that an organization's audit process is effective and efficient. It outlines the rules that define the scope of the audit and the criteria for evaluating compliance with the policies and procedures of the organization. The purpose of an audit policy is to ensure that the organization's assets are protected, the financial statements are accurate, and that the organization is in compliance with legal and regulatory requirements.

In addition to policy rules, remediation workflows, and designated remediators, an audit policy may also include criteria for identifying exceptions, rules for handling confidential information, and procedures for reporting audit findings. By implementing an audit policy, organizations can ensure that they are regularly evaluating their operations to identify and mitigate risks and that they are complying with internal and external policies and regulations.

GMP Compliance Audit

A GMP (Good Manufacturing Practice) compliance audit is a systematic review of a pharmaceutical manufacturing facility, laboratory, or supplier to ensure compliance with regulatory requirements for the production, testing, and distribution of drug products. The audit is typically conducted by an independent third-party auditor, or by the company's internal audit team, to assess the level of compliance with GMP guidelines.

During a GMP compliance audit, the auditor will review the facility's documentation and procedures, inspect the manufacturing or testing areas, and interview key personnel. The audit will focus on a wide range of aspects including:

- Facility design, cleanliness, and maintenance
- Personnel training, qualifications, and hygiene
- Equipment validation and calibration
- Raw material and product testing procedures
- Quality control and quality assurance procedures
- Recordkeeping and documentation practices
- Complaint and deviation handling procedures
- Product labeling and packaging

The objective of a GMP compliance audit is to identify potential areas of non-compliance with regulatory requirements and to provide recommendations for improvement. The audit report will typically include a list of observations and findings, along with recommendations for corrective and preventive actions to address any deficiencies identified during the audit.

Self-Inspection

Self-inspection is a systematic and objective evaluation of a pharmaceutical facility's compliance with current Good Manufacturing Practices (cGMP) and other applicable regulatory requirements. It is performed by the pharmaceutical company itself to identify deficiencies and non-compliances and to implement corrective actions before regulatory agencies discover them during an official inspection. The goal of self-inspection is to ensure that the company maintains high-quality standards and that products are safe and effective for the intended use.

During self-inspection, the company should evaluate all aspects of its operations, including quality control, manufacturing, distribution, and storage. The company should also review its documentation, such as Standard Operating Procedures (SOPs) and Batch Records, to ensure that they are accurate and up-to-date. The findings of the self-inspection should be documented, and corrective and preventive actions (CAPAs) should be implemented to address any deficiencies found during the self-inspection.

Self-inspection is a key component of a company's Quality Management System (QMS) and should be conducted regularly to ensure continuous compliance with cGMP and other regulatory requirements. It is also a requirement for obtaining and maintaining a pharmaceutical manufacturing license from regulatory agencies.

These are the common items that are typically included in a self-inspection checklist:

- ***Personnel*:** Training, qualifications, hygiene, etc.
- ***Premises*:** Building condition, cleanliness, pest control, waste management, etc.
- ***Maintenance of buildings and equipment*:** Calibration, maintenance schedules, repair logs, etc.
- ***Storage of starting materials and finished products*:** Storage conditions, labeling, segregation, etc.
- ***Equipment*:** Maintenance, calibration, cleaning, sanitation, validation, etc.
- ***Production and in-process controls*:** Batch records, standard operating procedures, product sampling, labeling, etc.

- ***Quality control***: Laboratory operations, analytical testing, the release of finished products, etc.
- ***Documentation***: Recordkeeping, document control, change control, etc.
- ***Sanitation and hygiene:*** Cleaning schedules, cleaning procedures, hand-washing facilities, etc.
- ***Validation and revalidation programs***: Validation plans, revalidation schedules, etc.
- ***Calibration of instruments or measurement systems***: Calibration schedules, calibration logs, etc.
- ***Recall procedures***: Recall procedures, mock recall exercises, etc.
- ***Complaints management***: Complaint handling procedures, investigation logs, etc.
- ***Labels control***: Labeling procedures, label storage, label control logs, etc.
- ***Results of previous self-inspections and any corrective steps are taken***: Previous inspection reports, corrective and preventive action (CAPA) plans, etc.

Types of Quality Audits

There are several types of quality audits, including:

1. ***Internal audits***: These audits are conducted by an organization's internal auditors to assess the effectiveness of the quality management system and compliance with regulations and standards.
2. ***External audits***: These audits are conducted by an independent third-party auditor, such as a regulatory agency or certification body, to assess compliance with regulations and standards.
3. ***Supplier audits***: These audits are conducted by an organization to assess the quality management system of its suppliers.
4. ***Process audits***: These audits are conducted to evaluate the effectiveness and efficiency of specific processes within an organization.
5. ***Product audits***: These audits are conducted to evaluate the quality of a specific product or service.
6. ***System audits***: These audits are conducted to evaluate the effectiveness of an organization's entire quality management system.

Internal Audit

Internal (First Party) Audits: An internal audit is a type of quality audit that is conducted by an organization's internal audit team or department. The purpose of an internal audit is to assess the organization's quality management system (QMS) and to identify areas for improvement.

Internal audits are typically conducted regularly and are based on a pre-determined audit schedule. The internal audit team will review the organization's QMS documentation, processes, procedures, and records to ensure that they comply with relevant standards and regulations.

Internal audits can also be used to assess the effectiveness of corrective actions that have been taken in response to previous audit findings. The internal audit team will report their findings to management, and recommendations for improvement will be made.

Internal audits can be beneficial for an organization as they help to identify areas for improvement and ensure that the QMS is functioning effectively. It also helps the organization to be prepared for external audits by regulatory authorities.

Internal (First Party) Audits are conducted by the organization's personnel to evaluate and improve the effectiveness of their quality systems. The key purposes of internal audits are:

1. To identify and address minor problems and errors before they become major issues or are discovered by a third party.
2. To ensure that adequate quality systems are maintained and that the organization is complying with relevant regulations and standards.
3. To achieve consistency between manufacturing and testing facilities.
4. To identify and correct problems internally before a regulatory inspection occurs.

The internal audit system should be designed to assess the activities carried out by different departments and the documents maintained by these departments. The implementation of an internal audit system should include the following steps:

1. Constitute a small team of experts who are familiar with the organization's quality systems and regulations.
2. Provide initial training to the audit team on the audit process and the organization's quality systems.
3. Fix the audit schedule (usually conducted at least once every six months).
4. Report the audit findings to top management and identify corrective actions that need to be taken.
5. Repeat the audit as per the preplanned schedule.

By conducting internal audits, organizations can improve their quality systems, ensure compliance with regulations and standards, and prevent potential issues from becoming major problems.

***External Audit (2nd Party)*:** An external audit is an independent examination of an organization's financial statements and operations conducted by an external auditor who is not a part of the organization being audited. The primary purpose of an external audit is to assure stakeholders that the financial statements of the organization are free from material misstatements and fairly represent the financial position, performance, and cash flows of the organization.

External audits are typically conducted by certified public accountants (CPAs) who are licensed to provide independent audits. These auditors follow generally accepted auditing standards (GAAS) and use their professional judgment to assess the organization's financial records, internal controls, and compliance with applicable laws and regulations.

The external auditor issues an audit report that summarizes their findings and provides an opinion on the fairness of the financial statements. The audit report is typically included in the organization's annual report and is made available to shareholders, lenders, and other stakeholders.

External audits are important because they help to enhance the credibility and reliability of financial information, which can improve investor confidence and help organizations access funding and capital. Additionally, external audits can help identify weaknesses in internal controls and provide recommendations for improvement, which can help organizations prevent fraud and other financial irregularities.

Purpose

- ***Confidence in the partnership arrangement*:** Vendor audits can help build trust and confidence in the partnership between the company and its vendors, by ensuring that vendors are capable of meeting the quality and safety requirements of the company.
- ***Ensuring that requirements are understood*:** Vendor audits can help ensure that vendors understand the quality and safety requirements of the company, and have the necessary processes and controls in place to meet those requirements.
- ***Enabling reduction of in-house QC testing of starting materials*:** By verifying that vendors have effective quality control systems in place, companies can reduce the need for in-house quality control testing of starting materials.
- ***Reducing the risk of failure*:** Vendor audits can help reduce the risk of product failures, by ensuring that vendors are capable of producing high-quality products that meet the requirements of the company.
- ***Confidence in vendor auditing*:** Regular vendor audits can help build confidence in the vendor auditing process, by ensuring that the audits are conducted consistently and effectively.

- ***Reduce the level of external auditing***: By ensuring that vendors are compliant with the company's requirements, companies can reduce the need for external auditing of their suppliers.
- ***External auditors have experience in GMP and are regularly audited by their certification body***: External auditors who are experienced in Good Manufacturing Practices (GMP) can help ensure that vendors are compliant with the relevant regulations and standards, and are regularly audited by their certification body to maintain their qualifications and expertise.

It is important to note that while there may not be a legal requirement for companies to conduct vendor audits, they can be an important tool for managing risk and ensuring product quality and safety. Regular audits can help companies maintain a high level of confidence in their supply chain and ensure that their products meet the required standards.

Regulatory Audit (Third party Audit)

A regulatory audit is a type of external audit conducted by a government agency or other regulatory body to assess a company's compliance with relevant laws, regulations, and standards. It is often referred to as a third-party audit because the auditor is not affiliated with the company being audited or its customers.

The primary purpose of a regulatory audit is to ensure that companies are complying with applicable regulations and standards and that they are operating in a safe and environmentally responsible manner. Regulatory audits can cover a wide range of areas, including health and safety, environmental compliance, financial reporting, and quality control.

Regulatory audits can be initiated by the regulatory body or may be required as part of a company's licensing or permit requirements. The audit process typically involves a review of the company's policies, procedures, and practices, as well as interviews with employees and inspections of facilities and equipment.

The regulatory auditor will issue a report summarizing their findings and providing recommendations for improvement, if necessary. The report may also include any findings of non-compliance and recommendations for corrective action.

Regulatory audits are important for several reasons. They help to ensure that companies are operating in compliance with relevant regulations and standards, which can help protect the health and safety of employees and the public, as well as the environment. They can also help to identify areas where companies can improve their operations and reduce risk.

In addition, regulatory audits can have legal implications. Non-compliance with regulations can result in fines, penalties, and legal action, and can damage a company's reputation. Therefore, companies need to take regulatory audits seriously and ensure that they comply with all applicable regulations and standards.

ROLE OF GMP AUDITS IN QA AND QC PROGRAMMES

Good Manufacturing Practice (GMP) audits play a critical role in Quality Assurance (QA) and Quality Control (QC) programs for companies involved in the manufacture, testing, and distribution of products regulated by government agencies such as the FDA, EMA, and MHRA.

The main role of GMP audits in QA and QC programs is to ensure that products are consistently produced and controlled by established quality standards. GMP audits are designed to evaluate a company's compliance with applicable regulations and standards, including the FDA's Current Good Manufacturing Practice (cGMP) regulations, and to identify areas for improvement.

In QA programs, GMP audits are used to verify that the systems and processes in place are capable of consistently producing products that meet the required quality standards. GMP audits are typically conducted by internal auditors or by external auditors contracted by the company. The audit process includes a review of standard operating procedures (SOPs), batch records, test results, and other relevant documentation. The auditor will also conduct facility inspections to verify that equipment is properly maintained, that personnel are adequately trained, and that environmental controls are in place.

In QC programs, GMP audits are used to verify that products meet established quality standards. QC GMP audits may be conducted internally or by external auditors, such as those contracted by regulatory agencies. The audit process includes a review of testing procedures and results, equipment calibration and maintenance records, and other relevant documentation. The auditor will also verify that personnel performing testing are properly trained and that testing is conducted in a controlled environment.

In summary, GMP audits play a critical role in QA and QC programs by ensuring that products are consistently produced and controlled by established quality standards. These audits help to identify areas for improvement and ensure that companies remain in compliance with applicable regulations and standards.

Benefits that are derived from Audits are given as:

1. Assuring GMP compliance.
2. Detecting Potential Problems.

3. Effecting Programmed improvement.
4. Increasing management awareness.

1. ***Assuring GMP Compliance*:** GMP audits are a critical tool for ensuring compliance with regulatory requirements. By conducting routine inspections, regulatory agencies like the FDA can assess whether manufacturing and control procedures conform to GMP standards. This helps to ensure that products are consistently produced and controlled by established quality standards.
2. ***Detecting Potential Problems*:** GMP audits can help to identify potential problems that may not be apparent to responsible production, QC, QA, or management personnel. Auditors can identify objectionable conditions and determine whether they are frequent or isolated incidents. This information can help to signal other GMP problems and can be used to proactively address issues before they become more serious.
3. ***Effecting Programmed Improvements*:** GMP audits can lead to programmed improvements by identifying areas for improvement and recommending changes to procedures, equipment, training programs, and documentation systems. By implementing these changes, companies can improve their overall quality management systems and reduce the risk of quality-related issues.
4. ***Increasing Management Awareness*:** GMP audits can increase management awareness of potential quality issues and help to ensure that they are taking appropriate steps to address them. By identifying areas of non-compliance and making recommendations for improvement, auditors can help to ensure that management is aware of potential issues and taking proactive steps to address them. This can help to reduce the risk of non-compliance and improve overall product quality.

Preparation of Audit

The preparation for an audit depends on the scope and may involve one or more auditors, with a lead auditor assigned and responsibilities agreed upon. It is recommended to rotate auditors periodically for internal audits. Contact with the auditee should be made well in advance to allow time for arrangements and initial information gathering. For customer or third-party audits, a primary contact within the auditee's quality assurance department should be defined. The lead auditor or inspector will communicate with the auditee to make arrangements and agree on the agenda before the audit. Relevant stakeholders should study the pre-audit questionnaire and seek clarification as needed. Previous audit reports and discussions with recipients can also provide valuable information. The audit agenda, including key reference documents and checklists, should be communicated and agreed upon with the auditee. The auditor should be aware of any sensitive issues or conflicts that may arise during the audit and handle them in a way that maintains a positive relationship with the auditee.

During an audit, the auditor should keep in mind certain factors that could potentially impact the relationship with the auditee. These include:

(a) ***Sensitive issues*****:** The auditor should be aware of any highly confidential information that should not be disclosed during the audit. Such information could be related to trade secrets, intellectual property, or other sensitive matters. The auditor should handle this information with care and ensure that it is not shared with unauthorized parties.

(b) ***Conflicts*****:** The auditor should be prepared to handle any conflicts that may arise during the audit. This could include disagreements with the auditee on certain issues or misunderstandings about the audit process. The auditor should remain professional and objective in handling such conflicts and work towards constructively resolving them.

(c) ***Relationship management*****:** The auditor should aim to maintain a positive relationship with the auditee throughout the audit process. This can be achieved by maintaining open communication, showing respect for the auditee's processes and procedures, and providing constructive feedback that can help the auditee improve their quality systems. The auditor should aim to build trust and respect with the auditee and avoid any actions that could damage the relationship.

- The audit should begin with an opening meeting where the auditor(s) are introduced to relevant staff and senior management representatives of the auditee, especially in the case of an external audit or inspection.
- The opening meeting also serves as an opportunity to explain the audit purpose, clarify the audit plan, agree on communication channels, and clarify any ambiguous responses in the pre-audit questionnaire.
- In the case of an external audit, the opening meeting is also an ideal time for the auditee to explain company rules regarding safety, taking photographs, the confidentiality of information, taking samples, talking with operators, making recordings, etc.
- The auditor should decide in advance whether to use a detailed checklist or rely on memory and experience by using an "Aide Mémoire."
- The auditors should have the freedom to spend more time on specific topics where compliance issues are becoming apparent and should use the "Aide Mémoire" as a guide from which they can deviate if a concern arises over an issue not covered by the checklist.
- During the audit, it is customary to walk through relevant parts of the facility to observe the operation firsthand, gather information, assess

the cleanliness and condition of facilities, and the risk of potential contamination.

- All relevant observations should be recorded clearly and concisely, along with supporting evidence. Any concerns should be discussed with the auditee as they arise to avoid surprises in the closing meeting.
- The selection of major areas that the audit should focus on starts with determining production, laboratories (both Quality Control and In-Process Control), storage (raw materials, intermediates, APIs, and packaging), transport and distribution, engineering and maintenance, development, and Quality Assurance.

In the closing meeting:

The importance of the closing meeting lies in the opportunity it provides for the auditor or audit team to present their findings and conclusions to the auditee's management in a clear and organized manner. An agenda for the meeting should be created and a brief written summary of observations should be provided.

In addition to highlighting areas for improvement with supporting evidence, it is equally important to emphasize positive aspects and commendable practices observed during the audit. The audit deficiencies should be classified to prioritize actions required by the auditee and their senior management.

Auditing Strategies

***Definition*:** It outlines the importance of having a clear direction for the audit, which helps to streamline the planning process and make it more efficient. The strategy document should include key decisions that will guide the development of the audit plan, such as the scope of the audit, the timing of the audit, and any specific areas of focus or risk that should be addressed. Overall, having a well-defined audit strategy can help to ensure that the audit is effective, efficient, and focused on the most important areas of the business.

The audit strategy is a crucial document that guides the direction, timing, and scope of an audit and is used to develop a targeted audit plan. The length of the strategy may vary depending on the size of the entity being audited, and unexpected changes may require alterations to be made with reasons documented.

The audit strategy is based on various factors, including the scope and characteristics of the engagement, reporting objectives, timing of the audit, nature of communications, significant factors directing the engagement team's efforts, results of preliminary engagement activities, knowledge gained from other engagements, and resources available for the engagement.

Considering these factors helps ensure that the audit is conducted efficiently and effectively, with appropriate attention given to areas that pose a significant risk or require more attention. The audit strategy provides a roadmap for the engagement team, enabling them to stay focused on the objectives of the audit and achieve the desired outcomes.

Audit Analysis

Audit analysis refers to the process of reviewing and examining audit evidence and data gathered during the audit process to determine the overall effectiveness of an organization's internal controls, financial reporting, and compliance with relevant laws and regulations. The purpose of audit analysis is to identify any potential areas of risk or noncompliance and to provide recommendations for improvements to management or stakeholders.

The process of audit analysis typically involves reviewing and testing a variety of financial and non-financial data, including financial statements, accounting records, transactional data, and internal control documentation. The auditor will evaluate this information to determine the adequacy of internal controls, identify any material misstatements or fraud, and assess the overall accuracy and completeness of financial reporting.

Audit analysis also involves assessing the effectiveness of an organization's internal controls, including its risk management and governance processes. This may involve testing internal controls related to financial reporting, as well as controls related to operations, compliance, and information technology.

Overall, audit analysis is a critical component of the audit process, as it helps to assure stakeholders that an organization is operating effectively, efficiently, and in compliance with relevant laws and regulations.

During the audit analysis, deficiencies should be identified and classified based on their severity. The classification is as follows:

1. ***Critical Deficiency*:** These are product quality or patient safety-related deficiencies that could potentially harm patients or consumers.
2. ***Major Deficiency*:** These are significant cGMP (Current Good Manufacturing Practices) deficiencies that do not directly impact product quality or patient safety but could affect the overall quality of the product.
3. ***Other Deficiencies*:** These are minor or isolated GMP deficiencies that are not classified as critical or major.

The auditors should provide the auditee with an opportunity to clarify and understand the evidence supporting the identified deficiencies. The auditor needs to identify what needs to be achieved to address the identified problems. In the case of second or third-party audits, the auditor should avoid being prescriptive on how to address the issues but can offer advice if requested.

Audit Report

The audit report serves as an important tool for identifying areas for improvement and for communicating audit findings to management. It is important to have a clear and concise report that accurately reflects the audit results and includes recommendations for corrective action.

There are two important reporting phases:-

(i) Preliminary reports during the audit

(ii) Final report to the management.

(i) Preliminary Reports During the Audit

The preliminary report during the audit is a draft version of the final report that is provided to the auditee during the course of the audit. It may include initial findings, observations, and recommendations, and can be used as an opportunity for the auditee to provide feedback or clarification.

(ii) Final Report to the Management

The final management report is the formal report that summarizes the audit findings, including any corrective actions taken or planned, and recommendations for improvement. It should be issued as soon as possible after the completion of the audit to ensure that any issues identified can be addressed promptly.

Audit Follow Up

Audit follow-up is a crucial step in the audit process that helps to ensure that the corrective actions have been implemented and are effective in addressing the issues identified during the audit. The purpose of the audit follow-up is to verify whether the corrective actions have been taken, whether they were effective, and whether they were implemented promptly.

Re-auditing may also be necessary to verify that the remedial actions have been implemented effectively and that the identified deficiencies have been addressed appropriately. The follow-up process should be documented, and the results of the follow-up should be reported to management for review and action.

Audit follow-up typically involves the following steps:

1. ***Review of corrective actions*:** The audit team reviews the corrective actions taken by the auditee to address the issues identified during the audit.
2. ***Evaluation of effectiveness*:** The audit team evaluates the effectiveness of the corrective actions taken by the auditee. This may involve reviewing documentation, conducting interviews, or performing additional testing.
3. ***Verification of implementation*:** The audit team verifies whether the corrective actions have been implemented promptly and are being sustained.

4. ***Reporting***: The results of the audit follow-up are reported to management and other stakeholders. This report typically includes an evaluation of the effectiveness of the corrective actions and recommendations for further improvements.
5. ***Follow-up actions***: Based on the results of the audit follow-up, management may take further actions to address any outstanding issues or implement additional improvements.

Overall, audit follow-up is critical to ensuring that the audit process is effective in identifying issues and that corrective actions are taken to address those issues.

Auditing/Inspection of Manufacturing Facilities by Regulatory Agencies

Regulatory agencies may conduct manufacturing audits to ensure that manufacturing facilities are adhering to regulatory requirements, good manufacturing practices (GMP), and other quality standards. These audits can cover a broad range of areas, including facilities, equipment, personnel, documentation, and procedures.

During a manufacturing audit, regulatory agencies typically review the manufacturing process and associated documentation to verify that it meets the established standards. This may include reviewing batch records, testing procedures, product specifications, and other documentation related to the manufacturing process.

The audit may also involve an inspection of the facility to ensure that it is clean, well-maintained, and equipped with appropriate equipment. The regulatory agency may also interview personnel involved in the manufacturing process to gain a better understanding of the process and identify any potential issues or areas for improvement.

The regulatory agency may also collect samples of the product being manufactured to test for quality and to ensure that it meets the required specifications.

Manufacturing audits are an important tool for regulatory agencies to ensure that manufacturing facilities are producing safe and effective products that meet regulatory standards. They help to identify potential issues early, allowing for prompt corrective action and preventing potential harm to consumers.

Those are some important reasons for conducting manufacturing audits. Here are some additional reasons:

- To ensure that products are being manufactured in compliance with regulatory requirements, industry standards, and company policies.

- To identify potential sources of contamination or defects in the manufacturing process.
- To evaluate the effectiveness of the quality control and quality assurance systems in place.
- To identify opportunities for process improvement and optimization.
- To identify training needs for personnel involved in the manufacturing process.
- To assess the performance of suppliers and subcontractors involved in the manufacturing process
- To identify potential risks to product quality and safety and develop strategies to mitigate those risks.

By conducting manufacturing audits, companies can ensure that their manufacturing processes are operating efficiently, effectively, and in compliance with applicable regulations and standards. This can help to reduce the risk of product recalls, improve customer satisfaction, and enhance the overall reputation of the company.

A Good Manufacturing Audit Requires: To conduct a successful manufacturing audit, several key factors must be considered. First, it is important to announce the audit in advance and emphasize that it is not intended to catch employees doing something wrong but rather to identify areas where they are performing well. A rating scheme should be used to classify any problems discovered during the audit, which will help prioritize corrective actions. When a problem is discovered, it is crucial to take action promptly and involve employees in the resolution process to increase their awareness and sensitivity to the issue. The auditors should be trained and knowledgeable about the process being audited and the auditing techniques being employed. Finally, careful planning and clear procedures are necessary to ensure that the audit is conducted effectively. The steps involved in planning and conducting an audit include selecting the process to be audited, deciding who will conduct the audit, determining the frequency of the audit, recording the audit schedule on a form, conducting the audit according to the schedule, documenting any problems discovered, informing all those affected by the audit results, determining and implementing corrective action, and monitoring the results of the corrective action. By following these guidelines, an audit can be a proactive effort to ensure that a manufacturing process is under control and committed to continuous improvement.

Conducting a good manufacturing audit requires careful planning, preparation, and execution. Here are some key elements of a successful manufacturing audit:

1. ***Clearly defined scope and objectives*:** The audit should have a well-defined scope and specific objectives to ensure that the audit is focused, efficient, and effective.

2. ***Knowledgeable and experienced auditors***: The auditors should have the necessary knowledge, skills, and experience to conduct the audit effectively. They should also be familiar with relevant regulations, standards, and best practices.
3. ***Thorough preparation***: The auditors should thoroughly review relevant documentation, such as SOPs, batch records, and test results, before the audit to ensure they have a good understanding of the manufacturing process.
4. ***Methodical approach***: The audit should be conducted methodically and systematically, following a pre-defined audit plan or checklist.
5. ***Open communication***: The auditors should maintain open and effective communication with the manufacturing staff during the audit to clarify any questions, gather additional information, and provide feedback.
6. ***Objectivity and impartiality***: The audit should be conducted objectively and impartially, without bias or conflicts of interest.
7. ***Comprehensive reporting***: The findings of the audit should be documented in a clear and concise report, which should include recommendations for corrective actions and a timeline for implementation.

By following these key elements, companies can conduct effective manufacturing audits that identify opportunities for improvement and promote continuous quality improvement.

Timelines for Audits/Inspection

The timeline should include key milestones, deadlines, and deliverables to ensure that the audit project stays on track and meets all requirements. When developing an audit timeline, it is important to consider the scope of the audit and the complexity of the project. A larger and more complex audit may require a longer timeline to ensure all aspects are thoroughly examined. Depending on the organization and industry, audit timelines can vary in length from a few weeks to several months. It is important to allow enough time for each phase of the audit process, including planning, fieldwork, reporting, and follow-up.

In addition to internal audits, external audits, and inspections also require timelines to ensure that all necessary preparations and activities are completed on time. These timelines should be communicated clearly to all stakeholders to ensure a successful audit or inspection. Overall, an audit timeline is an important tool for ensuring that an audit or inspection project stays on track and meets all requirements. It provides a roadmap for the project, helps manage resources effectively, and ensures that all deadlines are met.

The timelines for audits or inspections can vary depending on the type and purpose of the audit/inspection. Here are some examples:

1. ***Financial audits***: Generally, financial audits are conducted annually and cover the financial statements of the previous year.
2. ***Compliance audits***: The frequency of compliance audits can vary depending on the industry and regulations. For example, some industries may require monthly or quarterly compliance audits.
3. ***Quality audits***: Quality audits can be conducted regularly, such as monthly or quarterly, to ensure that processes and procedures are being followed consistently. Additionally, they may be conducted on an as-needed basis in response to identified issues.
4. ***Safety inspections***: Safety inspections are typically conducted regularly to identify and correct potential hazards. The frequency of safety inspections may depend on the level of risk associated with the workplace.
5. ***Environmental audits***: Environmental audits may be conducted regularly, such as annually or bi-annually, to ensure compliance with environmental regulations and identify areas for improvement.

In general, the frequency of audits and inspections should be based on the level of risk associated with the area being audited or inspected. It's also important to conduct audits and inspections regularly to ensure that any issues are identified and addressed promptly.

Benefits of an Audit Timeline:

1. ***Accountability***: A timeline provides accountability to the individuals involved in the project. It helps set ownership to different timeline stages, which can make the process of gathering new information more efficient and timely.
2. ***Timeline of Events***: A timeline can answer the questions of the "who," "what," and "when" of the event. Making this information visible to those involved in the project can help detect problems and prevent future occurrences.
3. ***Problem Identification***: A timeline can help identify problems that indicate system issues, operational issues, unusual or suspicious activities, or operator errors. This enables organizations to take corrective action and prevent future problems.
4. ***Evidence Gathering***: A timeline serves as a valuable tool for evidence gathering during an audit or investigation. It provides a clear and concise overview of the events and helps auditors or investigators determine if there are any irregularities or anomalies.
5. ***Communication***: A timeline can help communicate the findings of an audit or investigation to stakeholders. It can be used to present information clearly and concisely, making it easier for stakeholders to understand the scope and impact of the findings.

6. ***Continuous Improvement*:** A timeline can be used as a tool for continuous improvement. It provides a historical record of events, which can be used to identify trends and patterns. This can help organizations make informed decisions about process improvements and preventative measures.

Essential things to consider:

- Choose a secure location for storing the timeline and ensure it can be easily and regularly backed up.
- Gather all the valuable and necessary information relevant to the project to make the investigation more efficient. Review the timeline to ensure the accuracy of the data.
- Link artifacts to specific moments on the timeline to facilitate analysis of the "who," "what," and "when" of events.
- Share the timeline with relevant departments to keep the team informed and promote collaboration.

GHTF STUDY GROUP 4

Introduction

The Global Harmonization Task Force (GHTF) Study Group 4 has issued a guidance document on the regulatory requirements for medical devices. This guidance document provides detailed information on the regulatory requirements for medical devices in various countries and regions, including the European Union (EU), the United States (US), Japan, and Australia. The guidelines for regulatory auditing of quality systems of medical device manufacturers were developed by Study Group 4 of the Global Harmonization Task Force (GHTF). These guidelines provide recommendations and principles for regulatory bodies to assess and audit the quality management systems (QMS) of medical device manufacturers to ensure compliance with regulatory requirements.

The guidelines cover a range of topics including the audit planning process, the audit team, the audit scope, the audit methodology, the audit report, and follow-up activities. They emphasize the importance of a risk-based approach to auditing and encourage the use of objective evidence to verify compliance with regulatory requirements.

The guidelines also guide how to assess the effectiveness of a manufacturer's QMS, including a focus on continuous improvement and the importance of management commitment to quality. Additionally, the guidelines stress the importance of maintaining confidentiality and protecting the intellectual property of the manufacturer during the auditing process.

Overall, these guidelines aim to promote consistent and harmonized auditing practices among regulatory bodies and to ensure that medical device manufacturers are meeting regulatory requirements and producing safe and effective products for patients.

Their role includes developing guidance documents for auditing quality management systems, outlining competence criteria for auditing teams, and eliminating inconsistencies in auditing practices to address regulatory requirements for medical device manufacturers. The group began working on these documents in 1994-1996, at which time the ISO 10011 series and ISO 14011:1996 for environmental auditing were available.

The GHTF Study Group 4 guidance document covers several important topics related to medical device regulations, such as:

1. Quality management systems (QMS) requirements for medical devices.
2. Pre-market regulatory requirements, including product classification and conformity assessment.
3. Post-market regulatory requirements, including vigilance reporting and adverse event reporting.
4. Clinical evidence requirements for medical devices.
5. Labeling requirements for medical devices.
6. Unique Device Identification (UDI) requirements.
7. Medical device software requirements.

The guidance document aims to help medical device manufacturers understand the regulatory requirements in different countries and regions and develop strategies to comply with these requirements. The GHTF Study Group 4 guidance document is a valuable resource for anyone involved in the development, manufacture, and distribution of medical devices.

The Study Group 4 documents guide regulators and auditing organizations performing audits of quality management systems for medical device manufacturers using a process approach to quality management system requirements, such as ISO 13485:2003 and 21 CFR Part 820. By incorporating quality management system requirements into regulations applicable to medical device manufacturers, there is an opportunity for global harmonization. These guidelines can be used by regulators when establishing regulatory systems for medical devices. Note that "audit" in these guidelines refers to a regulatory audit. The potential benefits of following these guidelines include providing a high level of assurance for patients and users that safe and effective devices will be available, and independent, reliable, objective evaluation of compliance with regulatory requirements of the manufacturer's quality management system. If satisfactory, the audit results can serve as evidence of compliance with regulatory requirements needed to market devices.

Purpose of Study Group SG4

The purpose of the GHTF (Global Harmonization Task Force) Study Group 4 is to develop and promote international harmonization of regulatory requirements for medical devices. Specifically, Study Group 4 focuses on the development of harmonized principles for auditing medical device manufacturer's quality management systems (QMS). The group aims to ensure that the auditing practices used by regulatory audit organizations, auditors, and medical device manufacturers are consistent, efficient, and effective in verifying compliance with applicable regulatory requirements. By promoting harmonization, Study Group 4 seeks to eliminate duplication of effort and reduce regulatory burdens for both industry and regulators, while also ensuring that medical devices meet the highest standards of quality and safety.

STUDY GROUP 4 MEMBERSHIP

The membership of Study Group 4 includes regulatory and industry bodies from different countries.

Specifically, the United States has 2 regulatory bodies and 1 industrial body; Canada has 1 regulatory body and 1 industry body; Australia has 1 regulatory body; the European Union has 2 regulatory bodies, 3 industry bodies, and 2 Notified Bodies; Japan has 2 regulatory bodies and 1 industry body; and Taiwan has 1 regulatory body (as an AHWP liaison).

Scope

The scope of the GHTF Study Group 4 guidance document is to guide auditing organizations that are responsible for auditing the quality management systems (QMS) of medical device manufacturers. The document covers all aspects of the audit process, including planning, conducting, and documenting the audit, as well as follow-up actions that may be necessary to address any deficiencies identified during the audit. The guidance also includes criteria for the competence of the audit team, ensuring that they possess the necessary skills, knowledge, and experience to conduct effective audits. The document is intended to promote consistency and effectiveness in the auditing process, thereby contributing to the overall quality and safety of medical devices.

Rationale

The rationale behind the GHTF Study Group 4 guidance document is to promote consistency in the auditing of medical device manufacturer's quality management systems. Consistency in auditing is essential for achieving harmonization and mutual acceptance of audit results. When auditing organizations follow a consistent and harmonized approach to auditing, it helps to eliminate differences in the interpretation and application of regulatory requirements, reducing the potential for confusion and errors in the auditing process. Mutual acceptance of audit results can also help to reduce the burden on medical device manufacturers, as they will not have to undergo multiple audits by different regulatory authorities. Additionally, consistent auditing practices promote transparency and accountability, allowing regulatory authorities to ensure that medical device manufacturers are meeting applicable regulatory requirements and producing safe and effective medical devices. Overall, the GHTF Study Group 4 guidance document provides a framework for consistent, effective, and efficient auditing practices, thereby promoting the safety and quality of medical devices on a global scale.

The list of GHTF documents provided includes both archived and final versions of guidelines for regulatory auditing of quality management systems of medical device manufacturers developed by Study Group 4. The purpose of these documents is to provide guidance and harmonized principles for the auditing process of medical device manufacturer's quality management systems.

The archived documents include GHTF/SG4/N28R4:2008, GHTF/SG4/N30:2010, GHTF-SG4-N33 R16, GHTF-SG4-(00)3, GHTF/SG4/N30R20:2006, SG4(PD1)/N33 R13, SG4 PD N30R16:2005, GHTF/SG4/N26R1:2001, GHTF/SG4/N(99)24R3:2002, GHTF.SG4.(99)14, and GHTF.SG4.(99)28. These documents cover topics such as general requirements, training requirements for auditors, regulatory auditing strategy, audit language requirements, multiple-site auditing, and audits of manufacturer control of suppliers.

The final documents include GHTF/SG4/N83:2010 and GHTF/SG4/N84:2010, which cover Part 4: Multiple Site Auditing and Part 5: Audits of Manufacturer Control of Suppliers, respectively. These final documents provide updated guidance and harmonized principles for the auditing process of medical device manufacturer's quality management systems.

Overall, these GHTF Study Group 4 documents are important resources for regulatory audit organizations, auditors, and medical device manufacturers to ensure consistency and eliminate duplication of effort in auditing practices, promoting the safety and quality of medical devices on a global scale.

ISO 13485

ISO 13485 is an international standard that specifies requirements for a quality management system (QMS) for medical devices. It was first published in 1996 and is now in its third edition, published in 2016.

The standard is designed to ensure that medical devices are consistently produced and controlled according to applicable regulatory requirements. It covers the entire lifecycle of a medical device, from design and development to production, installation, and servicing.

ISO 13485 is intended to be used by organizations involved in the design, production, and distribution of medical devices, as well as by regulatory agencies and other stakeholders. It is a voluntary standard, but compliance with its requirements can help organizations demonstrate their commitment to quality and regulatory compliance.

Some of the key requirements of ISO 13485 include:

- Establishing and maintaining a quality management system that is appropriate for the organization and the type of medical devices being produced
- Identifying and managing risks associated with the use of medical devices
- Ensuring that all personnel are properly trained and competent to carry out their roles
- Documenting and controlling all aspects of the design and development process
- Ensuring that all medical devices are properly labeled, packaged, and stored
- Establishing procedures for monitoring and measuring the performance of the quality management system and taking corrective actions when necessary.

ISO 13485 is similar in many ways to the ISO 9001 standard for general quality management systems, but it includes additional requirements specific to the medical device industry.

Benefits of Implementing ISO 13485. Here's a More Detailed Explanation of Each Benefit:

1. ***Suitable for both small and large organizations*:** ISO 13485 is a flexible standard that can be adapted to the size and complexity of an organization, making it suitable for both small and large organizations.
2. ***Better internal management*:** Implementing ISO 13485 requires an organization to establish and maintain a quality management system, which can lead to better internal management practices and improved communication between departments.
3. ***Less wastage*:** By identifying and managing risks associated with the use of medical devices, ISO 13485 can help organizations reduce wastage and improve efficiency.
4. ***Increase in efficiency, productivity, and profit*:** By improving internal management practices and reducing wastage, ISO 13485 can help organizations increase efficiency, productivity, and profitability.

5. ***Consistent outcomes, measured and monitored*:** ISO 13485 requires organizations to establish procedures for monitoring and measuring the performance of the quality management system, leading to consistent outcomes that can be measured and monitored.
6. ***Globally recognized standard*:** ISO 13485 is a globally recognized standard, making it easier for organizations to do business with customers and suppliers around the world.
7. ***Systematic process improvement*:** By establishing procedures for monitoring and measuring the performance of the quality management system, ISO 13485 can help organizations identify areas for improvement and implement systematic process improvement.
8. ***Higher customer satisfaction*:** By consistently delivering high-quality medical devices, ISO 13485 can help organizations improve customer satisfaction and loyalty.
9. ***Higher prestige*:** Achieving ISO 13485 certification can enhance an organization's reputation and increase its prestige in the medical device industry.

While the requirements for ISO 13485 are more comprehensive than the list you provided, the points you mentioned do align with some of the key requirements. Here's a more detailed explanation of the requirements specific to ISO 13485:

1. ***Adhere to the standard*:** Organizations that wish to become certified to ISO 13485 must adhere to the requirements of the standard, including establishing and maintaining a quality management system that is appropriate for the organization and the type of medical devices being produced.
2. ***Document what needs to be documented*:** ISO 13485 requires organizations to document their quality management system, including procedures, work instructions, and records.
3. ***Maintain what is required*:** Organizations must maintain their quality management system by ensuring that it is up-to-date and effective.
4. ***Have written procedures in place and ensure the effectiveness of the system that you implement*:** ISO 13485 requires organizations to establish and maintain written procedures for all aspects of their quality management system, including design and development, production, installation, and servicing.
5. ***Consider the risk factors in all activities*:** ISO 13485 requires organizations to identify and manage risks associated with the use of medical devices throughout the entire product lifecycle, from design and development to production, installation, and servicing.

In addition to these requirements, ISO 13485 also includes requirements related to customer focus, management responsibility, resource management, measurement, analysis, improvement, and regulatory compliance.

Certification Process

While the certification process for ISO 13485 may vary depending on the certification body, the steps you listed generally align with the typical certification process. Here's a more detailed explanation of the certification process for ISO 13485:

Phase 1: Initial discussion

During this phase, the certification body will have an initial discussion with the organization to evaluate its existing practices and determine the scope of the certification process.

Phase 2: Gap analysis

In this phase, the certification body will conduct a gap analysis to identify areas where the organization's quality management system does not meet the requirements of ISO 13485.

Phase 3: Certification documentation, training, and pre-assessment

Once the gaps have been identified, the organization will need to develop and implement a quality management system that meets the requirements of ISO 13485. This phase may include developing custom-written mandatory certification documentation, providing training to employees, and conducting a pre-assessment to ensure that the system is working effectively.

Phase 4: Certification audit

The final phase of the certification process is the certification audit. This audit is typically conducted by an independent certification body and includes a review of the organization's quality management system to ensure that it meets the requirements of ISO 13485. If the audit is successful, the organization will be awarded ISO 13485 certification.

It's important to note that achieving certification is not a one-time event, and organizations must maintain their quality management system to remain certified. Recertification audits are typically conducted every three years to ensure ongoing compliance with the standard.

The Latest Version of ISO 13485

The latest version of ISO 13485 is ISO 13485:2016, which was released in March 2016. This version of the standard includes several updates and additions, including:

1. A greater focus on risk management throughout the product lifecycle.

2. Clarification of management responsibilities and the need for top management to demonstrate leadership and commitment to the quality management system.
3. Clarification of training requirements and the need for ongoing training and competency evaluation.
4. Improved facility requirements, including the need for environmental controls, maintenance, and calibration.
5. Better alignment of design and development requirements to regulatory requirements.
6. More emphasis on control of suppliers, including the need to evaluate and monitor suppliers and ensure traceability of materials and components.
7. Requirements for complaint handling, including the need to establish procedures for receiving, evaluating, and investigating complaints.
8. Enhanced requirements for product cleanliness, including the need for validation and monitoring of cleaning processes.

It's important to note that ISO standards are periodically reviewed and revised, so it's a good idea to stay informed about any updates or changes that may affect your organization's certification status.

CLAUSES

These clauses appear to be referencing a quality management system standard, specifically the ISO 9001:2015 standard. Here is a brief description of each clause:

Clause 1: Scope

This clause defines the scope of the standard and specifies that it applies to organizations involved in the design, production, installation, and servicing of medical devices. The clause emphasizes the importance of a process approach and the need for continual improvement. It also requires organizations to comply with regulatory requirements applicable to their products and services.

ISO 13485 is a standard that specifies requirements for a quality management system (QMS) for medical devices. It outlines the requirements for the design, development, production, installation, and servicing of medical devices. The standard is based on the ISO 9001:2015 framework but includes additional requirements specific to the medical device industry. The purpose of the standard is to ensure that medical devices are safe and effective for their intended use and to facilitate regulatory compliance for manufacturers of medical devices.

Clause 2: Normative Reference

The purpose of Clause 2 is to list any normative references that are essential for the application of the standard. These normative references provide additional guidance or requirements that organizations must follow to meet the requirements of the standard. It's important for organizations seeking certification to the standard to also ensure compliance with the normative references listed in Clause 2.

Clause 3: Terms and Definitions

This clause provides definitions of key terms used in the standard. Clause 3 of ISO 13485:2016 provides definitions for key terms used throughout the standard, many of which are specific to the medical device industry.

- Active Implantable Medical Device: a medical device that is intended to be totally or partially introduced, surgically or medically, into the body or a natural orifice and which is intended to remain after the procedure.
- Active Medical Device: a medical device that depends for its operation on a source of electrical energy or any source of power other than that directly generated by the human body or gravity.
- Advisory Notice: a statement issued by a manufacturer to inform users of a potential problem with a medical device or of measures that should be taken to mitigate a problem that has already occurred.
- Customer Complaint: any written, electronic, or oral communication from a customer that alleges deficiencies related to the identity, quality, durability, reliability, safety, effectiveness, or performance of a medical device.
- Implantable Medical Device: a medical device that is intended to be totally or partially introduced, surgically or medically, into the body or a natural orifice and which is intended to remain after the procedure.
- Labeling: any written, printed, or graphic information appearing on or provided with a medical device, including the instructions for use, intended to be communicated to the user or patient.
- Medical Device: any instrument, apparatus, implement, machine, appliance, implant, reagent for in vitro use, software, material, or other similar or related article, intended by the manufacturer to be used alone or in combination, for human beings for one or more of the specific medical purposes.
- Sterile Medical Device: a medical device that has been subjected to a sterilization process and is intended to be sterile until the package is opened or the seal is broken.

Clause 4: General Requirements

This clause outlines the general requirements for a quality management system, including the need for documented procedures, control of documents, and control of records. Clause 4 is divided into two main subclauses:

4.1 General Requirements: This subclause outlines the general requirements for a quality management system (QMS) and emphasizes the need for organizations to document their QMS to maintain its effectiveness. It also requires organizations to comply with the requirements of the International Standard and any applicable regulatory requirements. The FDA's quality management system requirements, known as Current Good Manufacturing Practices (cGMP), are an example of such regulatory requirements.

4.2 Documentation Requirements: This subclause specifies the documentation requirements for the QMS, including a quality manual with the scope of the QMS, required procedures, and records. It also requires organizations to document any other documents that are necessary for the planning, operation, and control of the QMS.

It's worth noting that ISO 13485 is a standard specifically for the medical device industry, and as such, it includes additional requirements and considerations that may not be present in other ISO management system standards, such as ISO 9001.

Clause 5: Management Responsibility

This clause outlines the responsibilities of top management for establishing and maintaining the quality management system. ISO 13485 Clause 5 outlines the responsibilities of management in implementing and maintaining a QMS. This section contains six subclauses that cover the following areas:

5.1 Management Commitment: This subclause emphasizes the importance of management participation in the QMS. Top management is required to lead and be actively involved in the QMS implementation and maintenance process. They have key responsibilities such as establishing QMS policies, conducting regular reviews, and ensuring that resources are available for the QMS.

5.2 Customer Focus: Management is responsible for meeting customer requirements and relevant regulatory requirements.

5.3 Quality Policy: This subclause outlines management's responsibility for ensuring that the QMS applies to the organization and that it complies with all QMS requirements. Management also needs to provide a framework for establishing and reviewing the QMS, communicate it throughout the organization, and ensure that it is understood. The QMS must be reviewed for continuing suitability.

5.4 Planning: Management is responsible for ensuring that QMS goals, including regulatory and product requirements, are met and measurable. They must also maintain the QMS when changes occur within the organization.

5.5 Responsibility, Authority, and Communication: This subclause emphasizes the need for top management to define and communicate responsibilities and authorities related to the QMS. Documentation of each person's responsibilities is required, and top management must appoint responsibilities to staff and management to ensure QMS compliance. Internal communication is also the responsibility of management.

5.6 Management Review: This subclause stresses the importance of management review for maintaining the QMS and achieving improvements. Management review brings together all aspects of the QMS in the organization and creates cohesiveness.

Clause 6: Resource Management

This clause addresses the management of resources needed for the quality management system, including human resources, infrastructure, and work environment. ISO 13485 Clause 6 focuses on Resource Management, which covers the requirements for the provision of resources needed for the establishment, implementation, maintenance, and continual improvement of the QMS. This section has 6 subclauses:

6.1 Provision of Resources

Organizations are required to provide the resources needed for the establishment, implementation, maintenance, and continual improvement of the QMS. This includes resources such as personnel, infrastructure, work environment, and support services.

6.2 Human Resources

- Organizations must determine the necessary competence of their personnel and ensure that they are competent and aware of the relevance and importance of their activities to the QMS. • The organization must provide appropriate training, education, and/or experience for personnel that impacts the quality of the product. The organization must evaluate and document the effectiveness of the actions taken.

6.3 Infrastructure

The organization must determine, provide, and maintain the infrastructure needed to achieve conformity to product requirements. This includes buildings, workspace, utilities, equipment, and supporting services such as transportation and communication.

6.4 Work Environment

The organization must determine and manage the work environment needed to achieve conformity to product requirements. This includes the physical work environment (e.g. cleanliness, temperature, humidity), as well as the organizational culture (e.g. communication, ethics, safety).

6.5 Product Realization

The organization must ensure that appropriate resources are available for the product realization process. This includes but is not limited to, production and service operations, inspection, testing, and maintenance of equipment, and calibration of measuring and monitoring equipment.

6.6 Supplier Management

The organization must ensure that suppliers and contractors provide resources that meet the organization's requirements. The organization must evaluate and select suppliers based on their ability to provide products or services by the organization's requirements. The organization must also monitor and re-evaluate suppliers' performance.

Clause 7: Product Realization

This clause outlines the requirements for planning, designing, and producing products and services. ISO 13485 Clause 7 focuses on product realization, which includes the processes involved in planning, designing, developing, and manufacturing medical devices. This clause has six subclauses:

7.1 Planning of Product Realization

This subclause outlines the steps involved in planning for product realization. The planning should include defining the product requirements, establishing the processes and resources needed for production, and ensuring that all regulatory requirements are met.

7.2 Customer-Related Processes

This subclause emphasizes the importance of meeting customer requirements during the product realization process. It covers activities such as communicating with customers, obtaining feedback, and handling complaints.

7.3 Design and Development

This subclause covers the design and development of medical devices. It requires that a systematic approach is used and that design inputs, outputs, reviews, and verification and validation activities are documented and controlled.

7.4 Purchasing

This subclause outlines the requirements for purchasing materials and services needed for product realization. It includes supplier evaluation, selection, and monitoring, as well as ensuring that purchased products meet specified requirements.

7.5 Production and Service Provision

This subclause covers the actual production of medical devices and the provision of related services. It requires that processes are controlled and monitored and that records are maintained to demonstrate compliance with regulatory requirements.

7.6 Control of Monitoring and Measuring Equipment

This subclause outlines the requirements for controlling and monitoring the equipment used for measuring and testing medical devices. It requires that equipment is calibrated, maintained, and controlled to ensure accurate and reliable measurements.

Overall, Clause 7 focuses on ensuring that medical devices are designed, developed, and manufactured in a controlled and systematic manner while meeting customer and regulatory requirements.

Clause 8: Measurement, Analysis, and Improvement

This clause addresses the need for monitoring and measuring the performance of the quality management system, as well as implementing corrective and preventive actions to continually improve the system. Clause 8 of ISO 13485:2016 is focused on Measurement, Analysis, and Improvement. This clause is all about ensuring that your Quality Management System (QMS) is working effectively and that you are continually improving your processes. This clause contains four subclauses:

8.1 General

This subclause describes the requirements for monitoring and measuring your QMS processes to ensure that they are effective. It also outlines the need to monitor customer feedback, complaints, and nonconformities, and to take corrective and preventive actions when necessary.

8.2 Monitoring and Measurement

This subclause requires that you establish and implement a monitoring and measurement program to evaluate the effectiveness of your QMS. This includes monitoring and measuring your processes, products, and services, and analyzing the results to identify opportunities for improvement.

8.3 Control of Nonconforming Product

This subclause outlines the requirements for controlling and dealing with nonconforming products, including identifying, documenting, evaluating, segregating, and disposing of them. It also outlines the requirements for taking corrective and preventive actions to prevent further nonconformities.

8.4 Analysis of Data

This subclause requires that you analyze your QMS data to identify trends and opportunities for improvement. It also outlines the need to use this data to evaluate the effectiveness of your QMS processes, products, and services and to take corrective and preventive actions when necessary.

In summary, Clause 8 is all about ensuring that your QMS is working effectively and that you are continually improving your processes to meet customer and regulatory requirements. By monitoring and measuring your QMS processes and products, controlling nonconforming products, and analyzing your data, you can identify areas for improvement and take corrective and preventive actions to improve your QMS.

Practice Questions

MCQs

1. Types of quality audits includes______
   a. product and process
   b. management (system)
   c. registration (certification)
   d. All of above

2. When the auditor is an employee of the organization being audited, the audit is classified as an .... quality audit?
   a. internal
   b. external
   c. compliance
   d. Both A & B

3. The most comprehensive type of audit is the .... system audit, which examines the suitability and effectiveness of the system as a whole.
   a. quantity
   b. quality
   c. Preliminary
   d. sequential

4. _______ are the three parties involved in an audit that plays a role that contributes to its success.
   a. the supplier, the auditor, and the auditee
   b. the client, the auditor, and the audit
   c. the client, the moderator, and the auditee
   d. the client, the auditor, and the auditee

5. The time required and costs involved in an external audit are much higher as compared to internal audits.
   a. True
   b. False

6. Audit is a fact-finding process that compares actual results with ....
   a. specified standards and plans
   b. expected results
   c. premature results
   d. preliminary results

7. .... is also expected to provide the resources needed and select staff members to accompany the auditor.
   a. Auditor
   b. Client
   c. Internal auditor
   d. Auditee

8. For the benefit of the organization, quality auditing should only report non-conformances and corrective actions, but should not highlight areas of good practice.
   a. True
   b. False

9. If the auditor is not the employee of the organization being audited the audit is ....quality audit.
   a. Internal
   b. External
   c. Compliance
   d. Third-party

10. If the audit is carried out by the regulatory body or inspector is called .... audit.
    a. Internal
    b. External
    c. Third-party
    d. None of the above

11. Challenges that auditor's face are ....
    a. observation fear
    b. management intimidation
    c. fear of not raising an issue
    d. all of the above

12. The term audit is defined from the Latin word audit which means
    a. to inspect
    b. to hear
    c. to examine
    d. to investigate

13. What are the main types of audit
    a. external audit
    b. internal audit
    c. third party audit
    d. both a and b

14. ISO 13485 is established in the year.....
    a. 1996
    b. 1998
    c. 1979
    d. 1985

15. ISO 13485 is for.........
    a. medical devices certificate
    b. drug product
    c. biological product
    d. others

16. Before the audit is commenced, the auditor plans out the whole of the audit work is called___
    a. Audit plan.
    b. Audit note.
    c. Audit risk.
    d. Audit program.

17. Internal auditor is appointed by
    a. the management.
    b. the shareholders
    c. the government.
    d. the statutory body.

18. Phases of audit process include _____
    a. selection
    b. planning
    c. execution and follow up
    d. all of the above

19. The physical dimension of equipment and accessories – comes under which qualifications?
    a. Design qualification (DQ)
    b. Installation qualification (IQ)
    c. Operational qualification (OQ)
    d. Performance qualification (PQ)

20. According to WHO, QC is part of _____________ .
    a. GLP
    b. GCP
    c. GMP
    d. None of these

21. The scope of sanitation and hygiene covers __________ .
    a. Personnel
    b. Premises
    c. Equipment's
    d. All

22. High-level personal hygiene should be followed and observed by all those concerned with ___________ processes.
    a. Manufacturing
    b. Transporting
    c. Warehousing
    d. None of these

23. GMP ensures which of the following parameters ______ .
    a. Quality
    b. Safety
    c. Efficacy
    d. All

24. Which of the following departments holds responsibilities for Quality monitoring or audit?
    a. QC
    b. QA
    c. Production
    d. All

25. According to GMP all complaints must be reviewed according to written procedures.
    a. True
    b. False

26. Recall Operations can only be performed during the normal working day.
    a. True
    b. False

27. Written recall procedures are not necessary as long as everyone knows what they are doing.
    a. True
    b. False

28. Things you need to consider to ensure your premises meet GMP design standards…
    a. Design
    b. Layout
    c. Sanitation and hygiene
    d. All the above

29. All equipment should ……….
    a. Have an individual identification number
    b. Have identified cleaning and maintenance procedures
    c. Have maintenance fault logs
    d. All the above

30. GMP stands for
    a. Good Manufacturing Procedure
    b. Good Manufacturing Practices
    c. Great Manufacturing Protocol
    d. None of the above

Answers to MCQs

1. d	2. a	3. b	4. d
5. a	6. a	7. d	8. b
9. b	10. c	11. d	12. b
13. d	14. a	15. a	16. d
17. a	18. d	19. a	20. c
21. d	22. a	23. d	24. a
25. a	26. b	27. b	28. d
29. d	30. b		

Short Answer Questions

Q.1. Define audits and the role of GMP audits in Q.A and Q.C program.

Q.2. Define preparation of audit and conductance of audit.

Q.3. Short note on ISO 13485.

Q.4. Short note on Audit analysis, Audit report and Audit follow up.

Long Answer Questions

Q.1. Identify the steps involved in the preparation and conduction of the audit. Add note on audit analysis.

Q.2. Explain the process of GMP compliance audits in a pharma manufacturing company.

CHAPTER 4

Inspection

Inspection is a quality control activity that involves measuring, examining, or testing one or more characteristics of a product or service and comparing the results with specified requirements to determine whether or not it meets the established standards or specifications. The purpose of the inspection is to identify any non-conformities or defects and to ensure that the product or service complies with the desired quality standards. Inspection can be performed at various stages of the production process, from raw materials to finished goods, and can involve visual inspection, testing, or measurement using specialized equipment.

Inspection is a process of examining a product, service, or process to ensure that it meets specified requirements. The purpose of inspection is to identify any non-conformances or defects that may exist and to take corrective action to address them. Inspection can be conducted at various stages of the product lifecycle, from raw materials and components to finished products, and can be performed by internal or external parties.

Inspection can be done through various methods, including visual inspection, measurement, testing, and sampling. Visual inspection involves examining a product or component with the naked eye to detect any visible defects or irregularities. Measurement involves using tools such as gauges and calipers to measure dimensions and ensure they meet specifications. Testing involves subjecting a product to various stress tests or experiments to determine its durability and reliability. Sampling involves selecting a representative sample of products from a larger batch or population and inspecting them to determine if they meet the required standards.

Inspection is an essential part of quality control and assurance, as it helps ensure that products and services meet customer requirements and are safe for use. It can also help identify areas for improvement in the production process, leading to increased efficiency and reduced waste. Inspection can be conducted manually by trained personnel or through automated systems, depending on the complexity of the product and the required level of accuracy.

The Objective of Inspection:

1. ***Ensure compliance with regulatory requirements*:** Inspection is carried out to ensure that pharmaceutical manufacturing facilities are complying with regulatory requirements and guidelines. This helps to maintain the safety, efficacy, and quality of pharmaceutical products.
2. ***Enforce Good Manufacturing Practices (GMP)*:** Inspection helps to enforce GMP in pharmaceutical manufacturing facilities. This ensures that the manufacturing process is carried out in a controlled and consistent manner, with appropriate documentation and record keeping.
3. ***Authorize the manufacturing of specific pharmaceutical products*:** Inspection is also carried out to authorize the manufacturing of specific pharmaceutical products. This involves reviewing the manufacturing process and ensuring that it meets the required standards.
4. ***Monitor the quality of pharmaceutical products*:** Inspection helps to monitor the quality of pharmaceutical products in distribution channels, from the point of manufacturing to delivery to the end user. This involves sampling and testing of products to ensure that they meet the required standards.
5. ***Identify and address quality issues*:** Inspection helps to identify any quality issues in the manufacturing process or in the final product. This allows corrective actions to be taken to address the issues and prevent their recurrence in the future.
6. ***Ensure product safety and efficacy*:** Inspection helps to ensure the safety and efficacy of pharmaceutical products by verifying that they are manufactured by the required standards and guidelines. This is critical to protect the health and well-being of patients who use these products.

Pre-Approval Inspection

A pre-approval inspection is an inspection conducted by regulatory authorities before approving a new drug, medical device, or biologic product to be marketed. The purpose of the inspection is to evaluate the manufacturing processes and facilities of the manufacturer to ensure that they comply with regulatory requirements, such as current Good Manufacturing Practices (cGMPs).

The inspection helps regulatory authorities determine whether the product is safe and effective for use and whether the manufacturer is capable of producing the product consistently at the required quality level. The pre-approval inspection is typically conducted before the regulatory authorities approve market the product.

During a pre-approval inspection, an evaluation is conducted to ensure that the establishment complies with GMP requirements, particularly in terms of environment, quality management, personnel, facilities, and equipment. The inspection also evaluates the procedures and controls implemented in the manufacture of the product (pre-approval batches) to determine if they conform to the application commitments.

Additionally, the completeness and accuracy of the manufacturing and testing information submitted with the application are audited, along with the conformity of pre-approval batches with planned commercial batches (process validation protocol). Samples are collected for the validation or verification of the analytical methods included in the application. Pre-approval inspections are typically carried out for new chemical entities, drugs with narrow therapeutic ranges, new applicants, or manufacturers. These inspections involve an inspection team consisting of analysts and other specialists with expertise in the relevant areas, and they also include a review of the application.

Carrying Out

When carrying out a pre-approval inspection, it is important to focus on several key areas to ensure compliance and quality. These areas include:

1. ***Manufacturing process***: A thorough review of the manufacturing process should be conducted, with an emphasis on data verification to ensure accuracy and consistency.
2. ***Analytical documentation***: Relevant analytical documentation from the manufacturer should be collected, including a copy of the analytical methods used by the inspected laboratory.
3. ***Method validation report***: A method validation report should be obtained for reproducing the analytical methods used in the application.
4. ***Sample testing***: Samples should be tested by the methods described in the application to verify their conformity with the stated requirements.

By conducting a comprehensive review of these areas, the inspection team can ensure that the manufacturing process is in compliance with GMP requirements, the procedures and controls implemented are in conformity with application commitments, and the pre-approval batches are consistent with planned commercial batches.

Inspection of Pharmaceutical Manufacturers

The inspection of pharmaceutical manufacturers is an important aspect of ensuring compliance with GMP requirements. These inspections are typically carried out by government inspectors to assess the manufacturer's compliance with GMP standards. However, the guidelines and principles of GMP also have relevance in other contexts, such as self-inspection or internal audit of a factory, inspection by an independent person or group as a review of the quality system of a company in compliance with BSI or ISO, or audit of a manufacturer or supplier by authorized agents of a customer. In all cases, the objective is to ensure that the manufacturing processes and quality control systems are effective, reliable, and comply with the established GMP standards.

During an inspection, the regulatory authority evaluates various aspects of the manufacturing process, including:

1. ***Quality management***: The regulatory authority evaluates the pharmaceutical manufacturer's quality management system (QMS) to ensure that it is well-defined, documented, implemented, and maintained.
2. ***Personnel***: The inspection team evaluates the personncl's training, qualifications, and experience in their respective roles in the manufacturing process.
3. ***Facilities and equipment***: The inspection team examines the manufacturing facility's physical condition and its suitability for the intended manufacturing activities. They also evaluate the equipment and utilities used in the manufacturing process to ensure they are appropriate for the intended use.
4. ***Manufacturing process***: The inspection team evaluates the manufacturing process to ensure that it is consistent, reproducible, and capable of producing pharmaceutical products that meet the required quality standards.
5. ***Testing and analysis***: The inspection team reviews the laboratory facilities and testing methods used by the pharmaceutical manufacturer to ensure that they are appropriate for the intended use and are in compliance with the relevant regulations and guidelines.
6. ***Documentation***: The inspection team reviews the documentation related to the manufacturing process, including batch records, analytical records, and validation reports, to ensure that they are complete, accurate, and compliant with applicable regulations and guidelines.

The results of the inspection are documented in an inspection report, which is provided to the pharmaceutical manufacturer. If any deficiencies are identified during the inspection, the manufacturer is required to develop a corrective action plan to address them.

Objectives:

1. Assessing compliance with GMP guidelines issued by organizations such as WHO.
2. Verifying that production and quality control procedures are being carried out by data provided in licensing applications.
3. Assisting government inspectors in assessing manufacturers' compliance with GMP.

4. Providing a basis for self-inspection or internal audit of a factory.
5. Reviewing the quality system of a company in compliance with BSI, ISO, or other standards.
6. Conducting audits of manufacturers or suppliers by authorized agents of customers.

PROCESS

The process of inspection typically includes the following steps:

1. ***Planning*:** The inspection team will plan the scope, objectives, and activities of the inspection based on the type of inspection and the product being inspected.
2. ***Notification*:** The manufacturer will be notified of the inspection date and given a notice period.
3. ***Opening meeting*:** An opening meeting is held to introduce the inspection team, explain the inspection process and objectives, and to discuss the inspection plan and schedule.
4. ***Inspection activities*:** The inspection team will review documents, records, and procedures related to the manufacturing process and will also conduct physical inspections of facilities and equipment.
5. ***Sample collection*:** Samples may be collected during the inspection to verify the quality of the product.
6. ***Closing meeting*:** A closing meeting is held to discuss the findings of the inspection, including any non-compliances and observations.
7. ***Inspection report*:** The inspection team will compile a report of their findings, which will include recommendations for corrective actions if necessary.
8. ***Follow-up*:** In cases where corrective actions are required, a follow-up inspection may be conducted to ensure that the necessary improvements have been made.

The frequency and duration of inspections can vary based on the type of inspection and the compliance history of the manufacturer. Routine inspections are typically conducted every 1-3 years, while concise inspections may be conducted every 5 years. Follow-up inspections may occur within 6 weeks to 6 months of the initial inspection. Special inspections may be conducted as needed, such as in response to complaints or recall related to suspected quality defects in products.

***Frequency and duration of inspection*:** The frequency and duration of inspections can vary depending on various factors such as the compliance history of the manufacturer, the risk associated with the product being manufactured, and the outcome of previous inspections. Generally, the following factors are considered while determining the frequency and duration of inspections:

1. ***Compliance history***: Manufacturers with a consistent record of compliance with GMP through previous routine inspections are eligible for concise inspections. Such manufacturers may be inspected less frequently.
2. ***The risk associated with the product***: Manufacturers of high-risk products such as biologics or sterile injectables may be inspected more frequently than those producing low-risk products.
3. ***The outcome of previous inspections***: If non-compliance issues were identified during a previous inspection, a follow-up inspection may be conducted to monitor the corrective actions taken by the manufacturer.

The duration of inspections can range from a few days to several weeks depending on the complexity of the manufacturing process and the size of the facility being inspected. Generally, inspections are carried out during normal business hours but may be extended to include additional shifts or weekend work if necessary.

Inspection of drug distribution channels: Inspection of drug distribution channels is another important aspect of ensuring the quality and safety of pharmaceutical products. It involves evaluating the activities of manufacturers, wholesalers, distributors, and retailers of drugs to ensure that the drugs are handled and distributed in a way that maintains their quality and effectiveness.

The objectives of inspecting drug distribution channels include:

1. Ensuring that drugs are stored and transported in appropriate conditions to prevent degradation or contamination.
2. Ensuring that drugs are dispensed only by licensed and qualified individuals.
3. Verifying that the labeling and packaging of drugs meet the regulatory requirements.
4. Ensuring that drugs are not counterfeited or diverted to unauthorized channels.

The frequency and scope of inspections may vary depending on the risk level associated with the drug product, the size and complexity of the distribution network, and the history of compliance of the parties involved. Inspections may be carried out by regulatory authorities or authorized third-party auditors.

The Inspector Will be Expected to Inspect Establishments Such as:

During the inspection of drug distribution channels, the inspector will be expected to evaluate compliance with regulations and guidelines related to the storage, handling, transportation, and distribution of pharmaceutical products. Specific aspects that may be covered during the inspection include:

- Ensuring that the facilities used for drug storage and distribution are appropriate and meet the necessary standards.
- Verifying that products are stored at the appropriate temperature and conditions, as specified by the manufacturer or regulatory authority.
- Checking that proper documentation and record-keeping procedures are in place to ensure traceability of products.
- Ensuring that products are being transported and distributed by authorized personnel using approved methods.
- Verifying that the labeling and packaging of products meet regulatory requirements.
- Ensuring that counterfeit and substandard products are not being distributed.
- Investigating complaints and reports of adverse events related to the distribution of pharmaceutical products.
- Checking that the personnel involved in drug distribution have the necessary training and qualifications.

The frequency and duration of inspections may vary depending on the type of establishment and its compliance history. Inspections may be conducted on a routine basis or as a result of specific concerns or complaints. Follow-up inspections may also be conducted to ensure that corrective actions have been taken following previous inspections.

Methods of Inspection

Comprehensive/routine inspection: Comprehensive or routine inspections are typically more extensive and in-depth, as they are conducted when a pharmaceutical establishment is going through significant changes or when there is a need to evaluate the overall compliance with regulatory standards. On the other hand, concise inspections are typically shorter and focused on specific areas of compliance, as they are conducted for establishments that have already undergone previous inspections and have a proven track record of compliance with regulatory standards. The purpose of concise inspections is to confirm that previously identified issues have been addressed and that the establishment continues to maintain good pharmacy practice standards.

Follow-up inspection: A follow-up inspection is conducted to ensure that corrective measures have been taken following advice and notice given during a previous inspection. This type of inspection is usually carried out after a certain period to assess whether the corrective actions taken by the establishment have been effective in addressing the issues identified in the previous inspection. The frequency of follow-up inspections depends on the severity of the issues identified and the level of risk associated with the establishment's operations. The follow-up inspection report should include a summary of the previous inspection findings, details of the corrective actions taken by the establishment, and an assessment of the effectiveness of these actions.

Special inspection: Special inspection is a type of inspection that is undertaken to deal with specific complaints received about lapses or non-compliance with standards of professional practice. This type of inspection is usually unannounced, meaning the establishment being inspected is not given advance notice of the inspection. The goal of a special inspection is to investigate and assess the specific issue or complaint that has been received and determine whether any corrective actions need to be taken. Special inspections can be triggered by various reasons such as complaints from the public, non-compliance with regulations, or suspicions of illegal activity.

Investigative inspection: Investigative inspection is a type of inspection used to assess the performance of a new establishment whose scope of operation was previously unknown. This type of inspection is typically conducted when there is suspicion of non-compliance or violations of regulations, or when there is a need to investigate specific complaints or incidents. The inspection team will carry out a thorough examination of the establishment's processes, systems, and documentation to identify any areas of non-compliance or deficiencies. The findings of an investigative inspection may be used to inform regulatory action or to support the initiation of legal proceedings if necessary.

Frequency of inspection: The frequency of inspections varies depending on the specific circumstances of the pharmaceutical establishment being inspected. In general, inspections should be held regularly, with premises being inspected at least once every 12-18 months. If contraventions are often noticed, the inspection should be more frequent, such as every six months. For establishments with a good record of compliance, less frequent inspections may be needed. It is important to note that inspections can be conducted at any time, and unannounced inspections may be carried out to ensure that pharmaceutical establishments are always in compliance with regulations and standards.

References/information sources for an inspector for inspection:

- ***Existing national and international drug laws and regulations*:** These laws and regulations provide the legal framework for pharmaceutical operations and outline the requirements for good manufacturing practices (GMP), good distribution practices (GDP), good pharmacy practices (GPP), and more. Inspectors should be familiar with these laws and regulations and ensure that the establishment is complying with them.

- ***Codes of inspection*:** Some countries or regions may have their codes of inspection that outline the specific requirements for inspections. Inspectors should be aware of these codes and follow them as appropriate.
- ***Codes of professional ethics*:** These codes outline the ethical standards that pharmacists and other healthcare professionals should adhere to. Inspectors may use these codes as a reference when assessing the establishment's compliance with ethical standards.
- ***Health consequences of drug abuse and misuse*:** Inspectors should be aware of the health consequences of drug abuse and misuse, as well as the risk factors for drug abuse and misuse. This knowledge can help inspectors identify potential areas of concern and assess the establishment's efforts to prevent drug abuse and misuse.
- ***Available data on imports/exports/prohibited drugs*:** Inspectors should be aware of any import/export restrictions or regulations related to pharmaceuticals, as well as any prohibited drugs. This knowledge can help inspectors assess the establishment's compliance with these regulations and identify potential areas of concern.

Inspection Report

An inspection report is a document that outlines the findings of an inspection, usually conducted by an authorized body, to ensure compliance with applicable standards and regulations. The report typically includes information on the inspection scope, methods, and findings, as well as any recommendations or corrective actions required to address identified deficiencies.

The report should be detailed and accurate, outlining any issues found during the inspection, such as non-compliance with regulations, safety hazards, or other quality concerns. It should also include a summary of the inspection findings and any recommendations for improvement.

In addition to the specific details of the inspection, the report should also include information about the organization being inspected, such as its name, location, type of business, and the names of individuals who were involved in the inspection process. The report should be signed and dated by the inspector, and a copy should be provided to the organization being inspected.

Overall, an inspection report is an important tool for ensuring that organizations are operating safely and in compliance with applicable regulations and standards.

When conducting a quality control inspection, the inspector should document their findings in an inspection report. This report should include a detailed description of the inspection process, including the methods used to assess the product quality, the criteria used to evaluate the product, and the results of the inspection. The report should also contain a list of any deviations from the expected quality level, along with any corrective actions that were taken to address these deviations.

The quality control inspection report should be comprehensive and include all necessary information about the product and the inspection process. It should be written in clear and concise language and should be easily understood by anyone who reads it. The report should also include any recommendations for improvements in the quality control process, as well as any suggestions for further inspections or follow-up actions.

Overall, the goal of the quality control inspection report is to provide a detailed and accurate assessment of the product quality and to help ensure that the desired level of quality is being maintained.

Pre-production QC Inspection

Pre-production QC inspection is a quality control process that is conducted before the actual production of pharmaceutical products. This type of inspection is critical in ensuring the safety and efficacy of the final product. The purpose of pre-production QC inspection is to reduce quality risks by inspecting the inputs before they are used in production.

During pre-production QC inspection, samples are randomly taken and checked to ensure that the raw materials meet the specified standards. An experienced inspector inspects the products to ensure that the development team has communicated with the manufacturing team and that the equipment for mass production is similar to that of the prototypes.

Some of the key activities involved in pre-production QC inspection include checking the specifications of the raw materials, verifying that the manufacturing process is consistent with the product specifications, and ensuring that quality control measures are in place. The inspector also checks the cleanliness and hygiene of the production area, and whether the personnel have received proper training in handling the materials.

Pre-production QC inspection helps to identify and address any potential quality issues before they become bigger problems during the production process. By taking steps to ensure that the raw materials meet the required standards and that the manufacturing process is consistent with the product specifications, the risk of producing substandard or unsafe products is reduced.

In-process QC Inspection

In the process, QC inspection is a type of inspection that occurs during the manufacturing process of a pharmaceutical product. The purpose of in-process

QC inspection is to ensure that the product is being manufactured in compliance with the approved manufacturing procedure and meets the required specifications. This inspection involves taking samples of the product at various stages of production and testing them for their quality attributes such as purity, identity, strength, and dissolution rate.

In the process, QC inspection is critical for ensuring that the final product will meet the required quality standards. By conducting these inspections, any deviations from the expected quality can be identified and corrected promptly, minimizing the risk of producing a defective product.

In the process, QC inspection typically involves trained inspectors who are familiar with the manufacturing process and the quality requirements for the product. The inspectors may use a variety of analytical techniques to test the product samples, including chromatography, spectroscopy, and microscopy.

The results of the in-process QC inspection are recorded in a batch record, which is a detailed document that provides a comprehensive overview of the manufacturing process and the quality of the product at each stage. The batch record serves as a permanent record of the manufacturing process and is an important part of the documentation required for regulatory compliance.

QC Inspection in Production

QC inspection in production refers to the quality control activities that take place during the actual manufacturing process of a pharmaceutical product. It involves monitoring and testing the product at various stages of the production process to ensure that it meets the desired quality standards. This includes inspecting the equipment and facilities used in the production process, as well as the raw materials and finished products.

The purpose of in-process QC inspection is to identify any issues or deviations from the desired quality standards as early as possible so that corrective action can be taken before the product is completed. This helps to minimize the risk of producing substandard or defective products and ensures that the final product is safe, effective, and of high quality.

In-process QC inspection typically involves a combination of visual inspection, physical testing, and chemical analysis. Examples of in-process quality control tests include monitoring the temperature and humidity of the manufacturing environment, checking the weight and dimensions of tablets or capsules, and testing the content and potency of the active pharmaceutical ingredient.

Analytical Inspection

The analytical inspection involves a comprehensive assessment of the laboratory's compliance with GMP and specific aspects of laboratory operations related to drug product testing. The inspection includes reviewing the specific methodology used for testing the drug product, ensuring that standard operating procedures (SOPs) are complete and adequate and that laboratory operations comply with written procedures.

During the inspection, inspectors also assess the suitability of the specifications and laboratory procedures and their conformance with application requirements. The purpose of the inspection is to determine whether the data submitted in the application is authentic and accurate and whether the procedures used to produce the data contained in the application were followed correctly. Overall, the analytical inspection ensures that the laboratory is capable of producing reliable and accurate test results, which are essential for ensuring the quality of pharmaceutical products.

Quality System Requirements for National Good Manufacturing Practice Inspectorates

The quality system requirements for national good manufacturing practice inspectorates include several key components. These components are outlined in a document history and include an introduction, purpose, and scope. Definitions are also provided to ensure a clear understanding of terms used in the document.

The quality manual outlines the administrative structure, organization, and management of the inspectorate. Documentation and change control processes are established to ensure consistency and accuracy in all aspects of the inspection process. Records are also kept to document all activities and findings.

Inspection procedures are established to ensure thorough and consistent inspections are conducted. Adequate inspection resources are provided, including trained personnel, equipment, and facilities. Internal audits are conducted to ensure compliance with established procedures and identify areas for improvement.

The inspectorate has processes for handling complaints and issuing and withdrawing licenses and GMP certificates. The handling of suspected quality defects and rapid alert systems are also established. The inspectorate maintains liaison with the Official Medicine Control Laboratory (OMCL) and has processes for sub-contracting and assessing.

Finally, publications are provided to ensure transparency and communication of inspection findings to relevant stakeholders. Overall, these quality system requirements ensure that national good manufacturing practice inspectorates operate effectively and efficiently to maintain high standards of quality in pharmaceutical manufacturing.

QUALITY SYSTEM

These quality system requirements are designed for use by competent authorities responsible for Good Manufacturing Practice (GMP) inspections. The purpose of these requirements is to provide a framework for the development of a quality system for inspection services. By incorporating these requirements into their quality system, inspection services can enhance their credibility and willingness to accept national inspections. The quality system should cover all aspects of the inspection process, from planning to reporting, to ensure that GMP standards are met consistently.

A quality system is a framework of policies, processes, and procedures that an organization establishes to ensure that its products or services consistently meet or exceed customer requirements and expectations. A robust quality system provides a structured approach to identify, control, and improve quality throughout all stages of the product life cycle, from design and development to production, distribution, and post-market surveillance.

In the context of good manufacturing practice (GMP), a quality system ensures that pharmaceutical products are consistently produced and controlled according to established quality standards. A GMP-compliant quality system includes procedures for documentation, change control, deviation management, quality risk management, corrective and preventive actions, and ongoing monitoring and improvement of processes and products. The quality system is overseen by a quality unit, which is responsible for ensuring that all aspects of the system are effectively implemented and maintained.

PURPOSE

The purpose of having a common standard for quality system requirements is to ensure that adequate quality standards are maintained and to achieve consistency in inspection standards between GMP National Pharmaceutical Inspectorates. This is aimed at facilitating mutual recognition and confidence between those Inspectorates.

SCOPE

The scope of this document is to define the quality system requirements for national pharmaceutical inspection services involved in the inspection of Good Manufacturing Practice (GMP) activities and Good Wholesale Distribution Practice (GDP) of medicinal products. It applies to all competent authorities responsible for conducting these inspections.

DEFINITIONS

Quality System: A quality system is a set of procedures and processes put in place by an organization to ensure that its products or services meet specific quality standards and comply with relevant regulations and requirements. It includes all activities involved in ensuring that the product or service meets the desired quality level, from design and development to production, testing, and inspection.

Quality Indicators: Quality indication refers to a measure or set of measures used to assess the quality of a product or process. These indicators are often quantitative in nature and can be used to track performance over time, identify areas for improvement, and ensure that quality standards are being met. Quality indicators can be specific to a particular industry or product type and may include metrics such as defect rates, customer satisfaction scores, and compliance with regulatory requirements.

Pharmaceutical Inspectorate: Pharmaceutical Inspectorate refers to a government agency or department responsible for ensuring that pharmaceutical products are manufactured, stored, and distributed by established quality standards, regulations, and guidelines. The inspectorate may conduct inspections of manufacturing facilities, distribution centers, and other sites involved in the pharmaceutical supply chain to verify compliance with regulations and guidelines. The primary goal of the pharmaceutical inspectorate is to protect public health by ensuring that pharmaceutical products are safe, effective, and of high quality.

License: A license is a legal permission or authorization granted by a competent authority that allows an individual, organization, or entity to engage in a particular activity, subject to compliance with specific regulations and requirements. In the context of the pharmaceutical industry, a license may refer to a permit granted by a regulatory authority to a pharmaceutical company to manufacture, import, export, distribute, or sell medicinal products, subject to compliance with the applicable laws and regulations. A license may also refer to a permit granted to a healthcare professional to practice medicine or pharmacy.

QUALITY MANUAL

A quality manual is a document that outlines the quality management system of an organization. In the context of pharmaceutical inspectorates, it describes the various elements of the system for ensuring the quality of the inspection activities. The quality manual should be prepared and maintained by the inspectorate and should cover all the elements described in the quality system requirements document. It should also include quality system procedures that define the activities of the inspectorates and the arrangements for maintaining the quality system. The manual should reference the standards and guidelines used to develop it, such as ISO or EN norms.

ADMINISTRATIVE STRUCTURE

The administrative structure of the GMP inspectorate should be designed in a way that ensures impartiality and meets the objectives of quality management. The membership and operation of the inspectorate should be transparent and open to public scrutiny to maintain public trust in the inspection process.

The national inspection services are responsible for ensuring that the requirements of the relevant national legislation are satisfied. This includes ensuring that pharmaceutical manufacturers comply with GMP regulations and that the products they produce meet the required standards of quality, safety, and efficacy.

All personnel employed or used by the GMP inspectorate, including outside inspectors or subcontracted personnel, should not be subject to any commercial, financial, or other pressures that might affect their judgment. They should be independent of the pharmaceutical industry and must be assessed and licensed.

The system for obtaining fees should not improperly influence the inspection procedure. The fees charged for inspections should be reasonable and commensurate with the work involved. The GMP inspectorate should ensure that inspectors are not subject to any commercial, financial, or other pressures that might influence their judgment.

The GMP inspectorate should ensure that inspectors are not improperly influenced in their inspection of pharmaceutical manufacturers or persons assessed. They should also ensure that inspectors have not been involved in the design or maintenance of inspected facilities by way of any consultancy service or commercial arrangement.

Overall, the administrative structure of the GMP inspectorate should be designed to ensure the integrity and impartiality of the inspection process and to maintain public trust in the quality of pharmaceutical products.

ORGANISATION AND MANAGEMENT

The GMP inspectorate should have a well-defined organizational structure that enables it to maintain the capability to perform its technical functions satisfactorily. The organizational structure should be documented clearly, identifying its legal status, and how the inspectorate obtains financial support. An organizational chart should be created, showing clearly the responsibility and reporting structure of the inspectorate, including the relationship between its inspection and authorization (licensing) functions.

The Pharmaceutical Inspectorate should have sufficient resources at all levels to enable it to meet its objectives effectively and efficiently. Senior management should ensure that all personnel are competent and qualified to carry out their assigned duties and that they receive appropriate training to stay up to date with the latest regulatory requirements.

There should be a system for periodic management review of the quality system, which should be documented, and records should be retained for a defined period. The management review should cover all aspects of the quality system, including the organization and management of the inspectorate, the competence of personnel, and the effectiveness of the inspection process.

The GMP inspectorate should also have a clear description of the relationship between the inspectorate and other departments within the drug regulatory authority and other government agencies, where they operate as separate bodies. This ensures effective coordination and cooperation among various departments involved in drug regulation.

Overall, the organization and management of the GMP inspectorate should be designed to ensure that the inspectorate is adequately resourced and staffed and that its personnel are competent and qualified to carry out their duties. The inspectorate should also have a robust quality management system in place, with regular management reviews to ensure continuous improvement in the effectiveness and efficiency of its operations.

DOCUMENTATION AND CHANGE CONTROL

Documentation and change control are critical aspects of GMP compliance. The following are key points to consider:

Documentation:

- All GMP-related activities should be documented by a documented quality system.
- All documentation should be controlled and maintained to ensure that it is up-to-date and accurate.
- The documentation should be legible, understandable, and traceable.
- There should be a system for archiving and retrieving documents.

Change Control:

- A change control procedure should be established to manage changes to GMP-related activities.
- Changes should be evaluated for potential impact on product quality, safety, and efficacy.
- Changes should be reviewed and approved by authorized personnel before implementation.
- Records of changes should be maintained, including the reason for the change, the individuals responsible for the change, and the date of the change.
- There should be a procedure to evaluate the impact of the change on previously approved products.

Overall, proper documentation and change control procedures are essential for maintaining the integrity of the GMP system. It ensures that GMP-related activities are properly documented, and changes to these activities are evaluated, reviewed, and approved by authorized personnel. It also ensures that records are maintained and archived for future reference.

RECORDS

The Pharmaceutical Inspectorate should establish and maintain a system of records relating to its activities, which should comply with any existing regulations. These records should provide detailed information about the planning and scheduling of inspections, how each inspection is conducted, a description of the inspection process, follow-up activities, and recommendations to the body responsible for issuing licenses.

In addition, all records should be handled in such a way as to prevent their damage or loss and should be retained for an adequate period consistent with any legal requirements. It is essential to maintain the confidentiality of all records to the inspected party, which includes the pharmaceutical manufacturers or any other parties that are subject to inspection.

Proper record-keeping is a fundamental aspect of GMP compliance. It ensures that GMP-related activities are adequately documented, and records are maintained and archived for future reference. It also ensures that records are protected against unauthorized access, alteration, or destruction, and there are procedures in place for the retention, retrieval, and disposal of records.

INSPECTION PROCEDURES

During inspections, inspectors should follow established procedures and use appropriate tools and equipment to ensure accurate and reliable results. They should also document their observations and findings clearly and concisely, using a standardized format for the inspection report.

The inspection report should include a summary of the inspection process, including the scope, objectives, and methods used. It should also provide a detailed description of any deviations or non-compliances observed during the inspection, along with any recommended corrective actions.

The responsible person of the inspected company should be allowed to review and respond to the inspection report before it is finalized. Any disagreements or disputes should be handled fairly and transparently.

The Pharmaceutical Inspectorate should have a system in place to track and monitor corrective actions taken by the inspected companies to address any identified deficiencies. Follow-up inspections should be conducted as necessary to verify that the corrective actions have been effective and that compliance has been achieved.

INSPECTION RESOURCES

Personnel: The Pharmaceutical Inspectorate should have sufficient and appropriately trained personnel to carry out inspections effectively and efficiently. The staff responsible for inspections should have appropriate qualifications, training, experience, and knowledge of the inspection process. ¬ The inspectors should have the ability to make professional judgments and knowledge of current technology, including computerized systems and information technology. Individual training and qualification records should be maintained to ensure that the staff is competent and qualified to carry out their assigned duties.

Resources and Equipment: The Pharmaceutical Inspectorate should have access to the necessary resources and equipment to enable it to carry out its inspection obligations effectively and efficiently. This includes access to appropriate laboratory facilities, reference materials, and other specialized equipment necessary for conducting inspections. ¬ The inspectorate should have adequate access to transportation and communication systems to ensure that inspectors can effectively carry out their duties.

The inspectorate should also have access to appropriate software tools and information technology systems to support the inspection process, including data management and record-keeping systems.

Overall, the inspectorate should have the necessary resources, both in terms of personnel and equipment, to ensure that it can carry out its duties effectively and in compliance with relevant regulations and guidelines.

INTERNAL AUDIT

Conducting periodic internal audits is an important aspect of maintaining an effective quality system in the Pharmaceutical Inspectorate. These audits help to identify any gaps or areas of non-compliance and allow for corrective actions to be taken promptly.

Internal audit records should include the scope of the audit, the audit criteria, the findings, and any non-conformances, as well as any corrective actions taken. These records should be retained for a defined period to demonstrate compliance with the quality system requirements and to provide evidence of continuous improvement. The specific length of time that records should be retained may vary depending on regulatory requirements and organizational policies.

QUALITY IMPROVEMENT AND CORRECTIVE/PREVENTIVE ACTION

Quality improvement and corrective/preventive action are important components of a quality system in the pharmaceutical industry. Here are some key points to keep in mind:

Quality Improvement:

- The Pharmaceutical Inspectorate should have a system in place for continuous quality improvement of its operations.
- This system should include monitoring, measurement, analysis, and improvement of the quality system and the inspection process.
- The results of these activities should be documented and reviewed regularly to identify opportunities for improvement.

Corrective/Preventive Action:

- The Pharmaceutical Inspectorate should have a system in place for corrective and preventive action in response to non-conformances or other quality issues.
- Non-conformances should be investigated to determine the root cause and appropriate corrective/preventive actions should be taken.
- The effectiveness of these actions should be monitored and reviewed to ensure that the problem has been resolved and to prevent recurrence.
- All corrective/preventive actions should be documented and retained for a defined period.

COMPLAINTS

The Pharmaceutical Inspectorate should establish and maintain a procedure for dealing with complaints relating to its activities, personnel, or any contracted persons or organizations. The complaints should be investigated, and appropriate actions should be taken to resolve them. The procedure should be documented and should include the following:

1. ***Complaint handling process*:** The procedure should define the steps to be taken when a complaint is received. It should specify who will receive the complaint, how it will be documented, and how it will be investigated.
2. ***Investigation*:** The investigation of the complaint should be carried out promptly, thoroughly, and impartially. The investigator should gather all relevant information and evidence related to the complaint. The investigation should be documented, and the findings should be recorded.

3. ***Actions taken***: The Pharmaceutical Inspectorate should take appropriate actions to resolve the complaint. These actions may include corrective and preventive measures, such as changes in policies, procedures, or training programs. The actions taken should be documented.
4. ***Record keeping***: Records should be maintained of all complaints received and actions taken. The records should be retained for a defined period.
5. ***Feedback***: The complainant should be provided with feedback on the outcome of the investigation and any actions taken to resolve the complaint.

By implementing a well-documented and effective complaint-handling procedure, the Pharmaceutical Inspectorate can ensure that complaints are investigated and resolved promptly, and appropriate corrective and preventive actions are taken to prevent a recurrence.

ISSUE AND WITHDRAWAL OF LICENCES AND GMP CERTIFICATES

The Pharmaceutical Inspectorate should establish and maintain a system for the issue and withdrawal of licenses and GMP certificates, or for advising about the issue and withdrawal of licenses and GMP certificates. This system should ensure that license and GMP certificate applications are assessed and determined promptly. Additionally, there should be a documented system for taking appropriate action against a license or a GMP certificate, notably in the event of an adverse inspection report. This could include the suspension or revocation of a license or certificate or the imposition of conditions on their use. The aim is to ensure that only those manufacturers and/or wholesale distributors that comply with the principles and guidelines of current good practices and with the relevant legislation are authorized to operate.

HANDLING SUSPECTED QUALITY DEFECTS AND RAPID ALERT SYSTEM

The handling of suspected quality defects in medicinal products and the rapid alert system are important aspects of ensuring patient safety.

- The Pharmaceutical Inspectorate should have a well-defined system for handling reports of suspected quality defects in medicinal products, including procedures for investigation, evaluation, and follow-up actions.
- The system should include clear criteria for determining when a suspected quality defect warrants a recall and the appropriate level of urgency for each situation.

- The rapid alert system is a European Union system that allows for the rapid exchange of information between regulatory authorities about potential or confirmed risks to public health arising from medicinal products. The Pharmaceutical Inspectorate should be familiar with and use this system appropriately.
- The Pharmaceutical Inspectorate should maintain an updated list of all performed recalls, including the reason for the recall, the affected products, and any follow-up actions taken. This information should be readily available to relevant stakeholders as needed.

SUB-CONTRACTING AND ASSESSING

When sub-contracted personnel or experts are employed as part of an inspection team, they must be used appropriately and under the supervision of the GMP lead inspector. The lead inspector should ensure that any sub-contracted personnel or experts have the necessary expertise and qualifications to assist or advise in a technical capacity and that their involvement does not compromise the overall integrity of the inspection. The lead inspector should also be responsible for ensuring that any findings or observations made by sub-contracted personnel or experts are appropriately recorded and documented in the inspection report.

PUBLICATIONS

The Pharmaceutical Inspectorate may also publish guidelines, standards, and other documents related to the regulation and inspection of pharmaceutical manufacturers and distributors. These publications should be regularly reviewed and updated as necessary to ensure their continued relevance and accuracy. The Inspectorate should also ensure that these publications are readily available to the public and relevant stakeholders, such as healthcare professionals and industry organizations.

Model Certificate of Good Manufacturing Practices

A model certificate of good manufacturing practices (GMP) would typically include the following information:

1. Name and address of the manufacturing facility.
2. Date of the inspection and the date of the certificate.
3. Name and address of the regulatory agency that conducted the inspection.
4. Details of the manufacturing authorization or license issued by the regulatory agency.
5. A statement certifying that the manufacturing facility is compliant with the GMP requirements.

6. A statement specifying the scope of the inspection and any limitations or exclusions.
7. A summary of any observations or deficiencies identified during the inspection.
8. A statement regarding any corrective and preventive actions taken by the manufacturer to address the observations or deficiencies.
9. A statement indicating that the facility is authorized to manufacture the specified products for the intended market(s).
10. The signature and stamp of the authorized regulatory official issuing the certificate.

The specific format and content of the GMP certificate may vary depending on the regulatory agency issuing it and the requirements of the local or international market.

Documents need for GMP Certification: These are some of the important documents that are required for GMP certification.

A GMP Manual provides an overview of the company's quality system and GMP requirements and outlines the roles and responsibilities of personnel involved in the production, testing, and distribution of pharmaceutical products.

GMP Procedures describe the detailed steps to be followed for various operations involved in the manufacturing, testing, and distribution of pharmaceutical products.

A GMP Process Approach provides a systematic method for identifying and evaluating potential risks and hazards associated with each step of the manufacturing process.

Standard Operating Procedures (SOPs) describe the specific procedures to be followed for various operations involved in the manufacturing, testing, and distribution of pharmaceutical products.

Exhibits are additional documents and records that support the implementation of GMP procedures and requirements, such as equipment qualification reports, cleaning validation reports, and calibration records.

Sample Formats/Templates are standardized formats for various documents and records used in GMP, such as batch records, deviation reports, and change control records.

A GMP Audit Checklist is a comprehensive checklist that includes all the requirements of GMP and is used to evaluate compliance with GMP during an inspection or audit.

WHO GMP CERTIFICATION

WHO GMP certification is a process where the World Health Organization (WHO) assesses the compliance of pharmaceutical manufacturers with its Good Manufacturing Practices (GMP) guidelines. The certification is intended to assure the quality and safety of pharmaceutical products manufactured and sold in countries around the world.

The WHO GMP guidelines were first introduced in 1969 and have been revised several times since then to keep up with advances in technology and changes in the pharmaceutical industry. The guidelines cover all aspects of the manufacturing process, from raw materials and equipment to personnel and quality control.

To obtain WHO GMP certification, a pharmaceutical manufacturer must undergo a comprehensive inspection of its manufacturing facilities and quality management systems. The inspection is carried out by a team of WHO experts, who review all aspects of the manufacturing process and assess compliance with the WHO GMP guidelines.

If the manufacturer meets the requirements of the WHO GMP guidelines, it is awarded a certificate of compliance, which is valid for a specified period. The certificate indicates that the manufacturer is capable of producing high-quality pharmaceutical products that are safe for use.

WHO GMP certification is highly regarded in the pharmaceutical industry and is often a requirement for manufacturers that want to export their products to other countries. It is also recognized by regulatory agencies in many countries as evidence of compliance with international standards for pharmaceutical manufacturing.

With 191 member countries in the scheme, WHO GMP certification provides a solution for international commerce between these countries, especially for those without a developed regulatory agency that wants to import drugs. The basic principles of WHO GMP is similar to any established GMP requirement, and anyone following an established GMP procedure will automatically understand the principles in other GMP requirements such as Schedule M, CFRs, ASEAN GMP, etc.

WHO GMP requirements were developed by taking into account the principles in various GMP texts and considering the requirements of developing countries. These requirements are not for domestic use but for international trade. There are around 1000 WHO GMP-certified manufacturing establishments in India, with the West Zone leading, followed by the South, North, and East Zones.

New applications for WHO GMP certification are coming in every day due to an increase in exports of drugs, and India being a major exporter of drugs and pharmaceuticals globally. However, other purchasers like State governments, ESI, etc. have started asking for the certificates as preconditions, which is not necessary as WHO GMP certification is not for domestic use.

Certificates

These certificates play an important role in the international trade of pharmaceuticals, as they assure the importing country that the product has been manufactured by the WHO's GMP requirements and is safe for use. The Product Certificate (COPP) attests to the quality of a specific pharmaceutical product, while the Statement of Licensing Status provides information on the manufacturer's licensing status and compliance with GMP. The Batch Certificate confirms that a specific batch of a product has been manufactured in compliance with GMP and is suitable for release for sale.

To obtain these certificates, manufacturers must demonstrate compliance with WHO GMP requirements and undergo regular inspections. The member state issuing the certificate must attest to the conditions of the manufacturer, including authorization to market the product in the exporting country, regular inspections for GMP compliance, and authorized labeling.

INDIAN GMP CERTIFICATION

GMP Inspections in India

the Central Drugs Standard Control Organization (CDSCO) in India is the national regulatory body responsible for conducting GMP inspections of pharmaceutical manufacturing facilities in India. The CDSCO has its own set of guidelines for GMP, which are similar to the WHO GMP guidelines.

In addition to the CDSCO, various state drug regulatory authorities also conduct GMP inspections of manufacturing facilities located within their respective states. These inspections are conducted to ensure that the manufacturing facilities comply with the GMP requirements and maintain the quality of the products they produce.

Apart from regulatory inspections, some Indian pharmaceutical companies also seek certification from independent third-party organizations, such as the International Organization for Standardization (ISO), to demonstrate their compliance with GMP guidelines. ISO certification is not mandatory but is often seen as a mark of quality and can be beneficial for companies seeking to export their products to international markets.

The FDA conducts facility inspections in India for products intended to be sold in the US. However, these inspections do not include CTM (investigational drug) facilities or clinical-stage products. It's also worth noting that only a small percentage of Indian facilities have been inspected by the FDA, with about 100 facilities inspected as of 2021. In general, India relies on local inspectors to conduct GMP inspections and ensure compliance with regulatory standards.

GMP Regulations in India

In India, the GMP regulations are enforced by the Central Drugs Standard Control Organization (CDSCO) under the Ministry of Health and Family Welfare. The regulations are laid out in the Drugs and Cosmetics Act, 1940 and the Drugs and Cosmetics Rules, 1945. The regulatory requirements for GMP compliance are defined in Schedule M of the Drugs and Cosmetics Rules, 1945.

Some key elements of the GMP regulations in India include:

- Manufacturing facilities must be designed and maintained by GMP principles.
- Adequate and qualified personnel must be employed, and appropriate training provided.
- Procedures must be established for the receipt, quarantine, sampling, testing, and release of raw materials, intermediates, and finished products.
- Records must be maintained for each batch of product, including manufacturing and testing data, deviations, and investigations.
- The quality control department must be independent of production and responsible for sampling, testing, and release of products.
- There must be systems in place for handling and investigating complaints and recalls.
- Validation of critical processes, equipment, and systems must be performed.
- Cleaning procedures and validation must be in place.
- Stability studies must be conducted on products.
- Regular inspections by CDSCO must be conducted to ensure compliance with GMP regulations.

Non-compliance with GMP regulations can result in various penalties and enforcement actions, including suspension or cancellation of manufacturing licenses, product recalls, and legal action.

Practice Questions

MCQs

1. _____ are advised to coordinate with applicants on the exact timing of pre-approval inspections.

   a. FDA b. Regulatory bodies

   c. manufacturing industry d. all of the above

2. FDA conducts a post-approval inspection to _________

   a. ensures commercial-scale processes

   b. for an approved drug product

   c. to application commitments and CGMP requirements.

   d. all of above

3. _________is the purpose of an FDA inspection

   a. for an approved drug product conform

   b. to determine a firm's compliance with applicable laws and regulations,

   c. ensures commercial-scale processes

   d. performed to contribute to FDA's assurance

4. How many types of inspections are conducted by FDA?

   a. 5 b. 2

   c. 6 d. 4

5. Inspectors embedded in an organization, usually called an

   a. drug inspectors b. inspectorate

   c. committee d. none of above

6. _______ inspection is generally reserved for a new pharmaceutical establishment?

   a. Comprehensive Inspection b. Organizational inspection

   c. pre-approval inspection d. special inspection

7. ________ inspection can be reserved for establishments that have previously been inspected with a view of assessing standards of good pharmacy practice.

   a. Follow Up Inspection b. Concise Inspection

   c. special inspection d. all of above

8. _______ inspection used to assess the performance of a new establishment whose scope of operation was previously unknown.
   a. Follow Up Inspection
   b. Organizational inspection
   c. Investigative Inspection
   d. special inspection

9. _____ is undertaken to deal with specific complaints received about lapses or noncompliance with standards of professional practice.
   a. Special Inspection
   b. Investigative Inspection
   c. Concise Inspection
   d. Organizational inspection

10. The inspector should possess which of the following attributes
    a. Maturity, honesty, and integrity
    b. Ability to hold discussions with company management after inspection
    c. Commitment to hard work and long hours
    d. All of above

11. _____ inspection involves a complete assessment and testing of medicinal products to ensure that they meet the required standards.
    a. quality inspection
    b. Concise Inspection
    c. Organization inspection
    d. Follow up inspection

12. _______ is a method for root cause analysis
    a. Problem/incident detection and data collection
    b. root cause determination
    c. development of corrective actions and follow up
    d. All of the above

13. Which of the following are Quality improvement process tools?
    a. Brainstorming
    b. Decision matrix
    c. Flowchart
    d. All of the above

14. Cause and effect diagram is also known as
    a. Fishbone structure
    b. Ishwikafiagram
    c. Pareto analysis
    d. Both a and b

15. Common failures of CAPA implementation include
    a. Lack of examination
    b. Lack of agreement information
    c. Lack of communication
    d. All of these

16. Which one is not the most important of Root Cause Analysis (RCA)?
    a. RCA empowers you to identify corrective and preventive actions that are needed
    b. RCA helps you to identify the symptoms
    c. RCA enables you to identify the most essential problem that can be managed and solved by management
    d. RCA enables you to identify the least essential problem that can be managed and solved by management

17. Which is not one of the tools for Root Cause Analysis Identification?
    a. Fishbone Chart
    b. Matrix Diagram
    c. Five Whys
    d. Reframing

18. In Five Whys steps Cause defined by
    a. Direct Cause - Redirect Cause - Root Cause
    b. Symptom Cause - Problem Cause - Root Cause
    c. Input Cause - Process Cause - Output Cause
    d. Direct Cause - Indirect Cause - Root Cause

19. CAPA stands for
    a. Correlative Action and Protective Action
    b. Corrective Action and Preventive Action
    c. Contention Action and Precaution
    d. None of above

20. In ________ options below CAPA is not required.
    a. Audit
    b. Ineffective CAPA
    c. Customer Complaints
    d. Especial repair (level 3.

21. ______ are the types of CAPA.
    a. Minor and Major
    b. Main and Medium
    c. Minor and Main
    d. Medium and Major

22. SOPs Are used to ensure consistency in daily operations. What does 'S' stands for in SOP?
    a. Special
    b. Standard
    c. Safety
    d. Sustainable

23. Inspection is a Protective way of identifying hazards.
    a. True
    b. False

24. Apart from checklists, a safety ______ is important during an inspection.
    a. Log
    b. Record
    c. Mindset
    d. Guidance

25. Which of the following is an example of an intermediary?
    a. Sales representative
    b. Agent
    c. Consumer
    d. Producer

26. A producer decides to use an agent to get his products into the market. The producer is using______.
    a. Direct distribution
    b. Channel A distribution
    c. Intermediate
    d. No distribution

27. Which intermediary in the distribution process follows the wholesaler?
    a. Consumer
    b. Sales representative
    c. Retailers
    d. Agent

28. The five "W"s of Root Cause Analysis are
    a. who, what, where, when, why
    b. what, where, when, who, why
    c. who, who, who, who, who
    d. why, why, why, why, why

Short Answer Questions

Q.1. Defined inspection

Q.2. Write short note on Pre-approval inspection

Q.3. Summarize root cause analysis

Q.4. Write short note on Pre-approval inspection

Long Answer Questions

Q.1. Explain methods of inspection

Q.2. Describe the role of CAPA in pharmaceutical manufacturing inspection

Answers to MCQs

1. b	2. d	3. b	4. d
5. b	6. a	7. b	8. c
9. a	10. d	11. a	12. d
13. d	14. d	15. d	16. b
17. d	18. d	19. b	20. d
21. d	22. b	23. a	24. B
25. d	26. a	27. c	28. d

CHAPTER 5

Product Lifecycle Management (LCM)

Product lifecycle management (LCM) is the process of managing the entire lifecycle of a product from its conception, through design and manufacture, to service and disposal. LCM is an important business strategy for companies, especially in the pharmaceutical industry, to ensure that their products remain relevant, competitive, and profitable throughout their lifetimes.

LCM involves continuous assessment and management of a product, including making necessary improvements, changes, or modifications to the product, as well as monitoring and evaluating its performance in the market. The goal is to maximize the value of the product to customers, which may include expanding its indications, improving its formulation or delivery system, enhancing its safety and efficacy, and improving the patient experience.

LCM also involves strategies for managing product obsolescence, such as identifying when a product is reaching the end of its lifecycle and planning for its replacement or discontinuation. Effective LCM can help companies stay ahead of the competition and maintain a strong market position over the long term.

Annual Report

An annual report is a comprehensive report that provides information on a company's activities and financial performance over the course of a year. The report typically includes a letter from the CEO or Board of Directors, financial statements, performance highlights, and objectives for the future.

The purpose of an annual report is to provide stakeholders with an overview of the company's performance, financial health, and plans. These stakeholders may include shareholders, potential investors, employees, customers, and regulatory agencies.

The content and structure of annual reports can vary between companies, but most reports will typically include sections on the company's financial performance, operations, market position, and outlook for the future. Financial statements are a key component of the report, providing detailed information on revenue, expenses, profits, and losses. Performance highlights may include notable achievements or milestones, new product launches, and awards or recognition received by the company.

In addition to providing information on financial performance, annual reports may also highlight a company's commitment to corporate social responsibility and sustainability initiatives. This may include information on environmental initiatives, community outreach, and ethical business practices.

Overall, annual reports serve as a valuable tool for stakeholders to evaluate a company's performance and make informed decisions about investing, partnering, or doing business with the company.

Post-Marketing Reporting Requirements

Post-marketing reporting requirements refer to studies and clinical trials that are conducted after a product has been approved to gather additional information about its safety, efficacy, or optimal use. These studies and trials can be required by regulatory agencies or can be commitments made by the sponsor.

The FDA has a searchable database of information on post-marketing studies and clinical trials for drugs and biological products. Sponsors are required to provide a timetable of completion and periodic reports on the status of the study, including any difficulties encountered in completing it. They are also required to provide periodic reports on the status of clinical trials.

In addition, sponsors are required to report any serious risks associated with their products that are identified at the time of approval or after approval if new safety information becomes available. Sponsors need to fulfill these reporting requirements to ensure the safety and efficacy of their products and to maintain regulatory compliance.

Post-Approval Labelling Changes

Post-approval labeling changes refer to changes made to the labeling of a drug or biological product after it has been approved for marketing. These changes can be initiated by the sponsor or required by the regulatory authorities based on new safety information that becomes available after the approval of the product. These changes can include adding or updating warnings, precautions, contraindications, adverse reactions, or other safety-related information. The regulatory authorities have specific submission procedures and requirements for these changes, which the sponsors must follow.

Section 505(o)(4) of the Federal Food, Drug, and Cosmetic Act (FD&C Act) authorizes the FDA to require certain drug and biological product application holders to make safety-related labeling changes based on new safety information that becomes available after approval of the drug or biological product. This helps ensure that the labeling for a product accurately reflects the most up-to-date safety information for the product.

Section 505(o)(4) of the Act authorizes FDA to require safety labeling changes for the following products:

Section 505(o)(4) of the Act authorizes FDA to require safety labeling changes for prescription drug products with an approved new drug application (NDA) under section 505(b) of the Act, biological products with an approved biologics license application (BLA) under section 351 of the Public Health Service Act (the PHS Act), and prescription drug products with an approved abbreviated new drug application (ANDA) under section 505(j) of the Act if the NDA reference listed drug (RLD) is not currently marketed.

The provisions in section 505(o)(4) apply to prescription drug products with an approved NDA under section 505(b) of the Act, biological products with an approved BLA under section 351 of the PHS Act, and prescription drug products with an approved ANDA under section 505(j) of the Act, if the RLD is not currently marketed. The provisions also apply to products that are not marketed, unless the approval of the NDA, BLA, or ANDA has been withdrawn in the Federal Register.

However, section 505(o)(4) does not apply to nonprescription (over-the-counter) drugs approved under an NDA or ANDA or to marketed unapproved drugs. Additionally, the guidance does not address labeling supplements submitted voluntarily by an application holder. Application holders may submit labeling supplements for review at any time and without prior notification to FDA.

IMPLEMENTATION OF SAFETY LABELING CHANGES UNDER FDAAA

What is New Safety Information?

New safety information refers to a serious risk or an unexpected serious risk associated with the use of a drug that the FDA has become aware of since the drug was approved, since the risk evaluation and mitigation strategy (REMS) was required, or since the last assessment of the approved REMS for the drug. This information may be based on a new analysis of existing data or may be entirely new information that was not previously available. It is important to note that new safety information may lead to changes in the drug's labeling or prescribing information, including new warnings or contraindications.

How Does FDA Learn About New Safety Information?

FDA may learn about new safety information from various sources, including but not limited to, adverse event reports submitted by healthcare professionals, patients, or manufacturers, findings from clinical studies, epidemiological studies, post-marketing surveillance programs, and published literature. Once FDA becomes aware of the potential for new safety information, it may derive new safety information through various means, such as a new analysis of existing information, an assessment of the risks and benefits of the drug as it pertains to a new use or population, or information on the effectiveness of a previously approved Risk Evaluation and Mitigation Strategy (REMS).

How Will FDA Evaluate the New Safety Information?

FDA will form a multidisciplinary team to evaluate information that may be new safety information that should be incorporated into a drug's labeling under section 505(o)(4). The composition of the team will vary depending on the nature of the safety concern. The team's discussions and evaluations of the new safety information may include but are not limited to, presentations at internal FDA meetings, Drug Safety Oversight Board meetings, or Advisory Committee meetings. The team will evaluate the new safety information based on its potential impact on patient safety and determine whether it warrants a safety labeling change. More information about FDA's policies and procedures for drug safety issues is available in several Manuals of Policies and Procedures (MAPPs).

What Types of Safety Labeling Changes Could Be Required Under Section 505(o)(4)?

Under Section 505(o)(4), FDA could require drug manufacturers to make the following types of safety labeling changes:

1. Adding a new contraindication, warning, precaution, or adverse reaction to the drug labeling
2. Revising the recommended dosage or duration of use
3. Adding or modifying instructions for use or administration
4. Adding a patient Medication Guide or a package insert
5. Changing the drug's description or identity to ensure safe use
6. Other changes necessary to ensure the safe use of the drug

These changes may be based on new safety information that FDA becomes aware of after approval of the drug or biological product. The goal of these changes is to inform healthcare providers and patients about the risks associated with the use of the drug or biological product and to help minimize the potential for harm to patients.

How Will FDA Notify Application Holder(s) of Required Safety Labeling Changes?

After identifying the new safety information that should be added to the labeling, the FDA will send a notification letter to the application holder informing them of the safety labeling change requirement. The application holder of an approved NDA, BLA, or ANDA without a marketed NDA reference listed drug (RLD) will receive the notification and be mandated to implement the safety labeling changes, except in cases where the application's approval has been officially withdrawn through a notice in the Federal Register.

How Should Application Holders Respond to a Notification Letter?

After receiving a notification letter from the FDA regarding the required safety labeling changes, the application holder(s) must respond promptly and either:

- Submit a supplemental application with proposed labeling changes to reflect the new safety information
- Notify the FDA that they do not believe a labeling change is warranted and provide a detailed statement outlining the reasons why such a change is not necessary.

If the application holder disagrees with the FDA's determination that a labeling change is necessary, they should provide scientific and medical justification to support their position. It's important to note that the FDA may still require the labeling change even if the application holder disagrees with the determination.

When Should New Labeling Be Available

The FDA expects that approved new labeling reflecting the required safety changes will be made available on the application holder's website within 10 calendar days after approval of the labeling supplement or after the FDA's receipt of a changes-being-effected labeling supplement. The FDA also posts approved labeling updates on its website. However, the FDA understands that incorporating changes into printed material included in drug shipments may take longer than updating a website.

ENFORCING REQUIREMENTS FOR SAFETY LABELING CHANGES

Enforcing the requirements for safety labeling changes is an important aspect of FDA's responsibility to protect public health. Section 902 of FDAAA grants FDA the authority to enforce the requirements for safety labeling changes under section 505(o)(4). If the responsible person or application holder fails to submit a supplement within 15 calendar days of the date of a safety labeling change order or fails to initiate dispute resolution within 5 days, they will violate section 505(o)(4) of the Act.

In the event of non-compliance, FDA may take various enforcement actions, such as issuing warning letters, seeking injunctions, or pursuing other legal remedies available under the law. In addition, FDA may take regulatory action to remove the drug from the market if the drug poses a significant or unreasonable risk of harm to public health.

Lifecycle Management

Lifecycle management in the pharmaceutical industry refers to the process of managing a drug product throughout its entire life cycle, from its development, approval, launch, and commercialization to its eventual discontinuation. It involves various strategies to maximize the drug product's value, extend its patent life, and ensure its safety and efficacy.

Lifecycle management strategies may include:

- Developing and launching new formulations, strengths, or dosage forms of the drug product
- Seeking new indications or expanding the patient population for which the drug product is approved
- Conducting post-marketing studies to collect additional safety and efficacy data
- Implementing risk management plans to mitigate known risks associated with the drug product
- Submitting regulatory applications for approval of new indications or changes to the drug product's labeling or manufacturing process
- Acquiring or licensing new drug products or technologies to complement or expand the drug product's market position.

Lifecycle management is critical for pharmaceutical companies to maintain their competitive edge, increase revenues, and extend the patent life of their drug products. However, the strategies employed must be in line with regulatory requirements and must prioritize patient safety and healthcare provider needs.

Benefits of PLM

1. Reduced time to market: PLM streamlines the product development process, reducing the time it takes to bring a product to market.
2. Improved product quality: PLM ensures consistency in design and manufacturing processes, resulting in improved product quality and fewer defects.
3. Reduced prototyping costs: PLM enables companies to simulate and test products in a virtual environment, reducing the need for physical prototypes and associated costs.
4. A more accurate and timely request for Quote generation: PLM provides accurate and up-to-date product information, enabling more accurate and timely quoting of product costs and delivery times.

5. Ability to quickly identify potential sales opportunities and revenue contributions: PLM enables companies to analyze customer needs and market trends, identifying potential sales opportunities and revenue contributions.
6. Savings through the reuse of original data: PLM enables the reuse of original data and design components, reducing the need for redundant work and saving time and resources.
7. A framework for product optimization: PLM provides a framework for continuous product optimization, allowing companies to make improvements and updates throughout a product's lifecycle.

Phases of PLM

1. ***Conceive***: This phase involves the ideation and conceptualization of a product. In this phase, companies identify customer needs and determine the feasibility of a product.
2. ***Design***: In this phase, the product is designed, tested, and validated. The design phase also includes activities such as prototyping and simulation.
3. ***Realize***: In this phase, the product is manufactured, sold, and delivered to customers. This phase also includes activities such as procurement, production, and supply chain management.
4. ***Service***: In this phase, the product is used by customers, and companies provide services such as maintenance, repair, and support. The service phase also includes activities such as product phase-out, retirement, recycling, and disposal.

PHASE 1: CONCEIVE [IMAGINE, SPECIFY, PLAN, INNOVATE]

The Conceive phase is the first phase of PLM, which involves the initial planning and conceptualization of a product. During this phase, the product idea is identified, and its feasibility is evaluated. The following are the key activities that take place during the Conceive phase:

1. ***Imagine***: This involves generating product ideas through brainstorming, market research, customer feedback, and other sources.
2. ***Specify***: In this step, the product requirements and specifications are defined. This includes the product features, functions, performance, and other technical requirements.
3. ***Plan***: A project plan is developed for the product development process. The plan includes a timeline, budget, resource allocation, and risk assessment.
4. ***Innovate***: This step involves exploring new technologies, materials, and design concepts to create innovative products that meet customer needs.

The Conceive phase is critical for the success of the product development process, as it sets the foundation for the subsequent phases of PLM. By thoroughly defining the product requirements and specifications, the team can ensure that the product meets the customer's needs and expectations.

PHASE 2: DESIGN [DESCRIBE, DEFINE, DEVELOP, TEST, ANALYZE AND VALIDATE]

The Design phase of PLM involves the detailed design and development of the product, progressing from the conception phase. This phase includes:

1. ***Describe*:** In this stage, the product is described, and the design requirements are established. The design team defines the product's function, features, and appearance.
2. ***Define*:** In this stage, the detailed design process begins. The design team starts with the product's specifications and develops a complete design plan, including material selection, component selection, and manufacturing processes.
3. ***Develop*:** In this stage, the design plan is implemented, and prototypes of the product are produced. The design team works to refine the design to ensure it meets the product's requirements.
4. ***Test*:** In this stage, the prototypes are tested to ensure they meet the design specifications. The design team performs various tests, including stress tests, load tests, and environmental tests.
5. ***Analyze*:** In this stage, the design team analyzes the test results to determine if any changes need to be made to the product design. The team evaluates the performance of the product and determines whether it meets the desired level of quality.
6. ***Validate*:** In this stage, the final design is validated. The design team checks the product's performance, functionality, and reliability. If the product meets the desired level of quality, the design is approved for production.

The main tool used for the Design phase of PLM is CAD (Computer-Aided Design) software. This software allows designers to create and modify 2D and 3D models of the product, enabling them to visualize the product design and identify potential issues early on in the design process. Additionally, CAE (Computer-Aided Engineering) software is used to perform tasks such as stress analysis, FEA (Finite Element Analysis), kinematics, computational fluid dynamics (CFD), and mechanical event simulation (MES). These tools help designers optimize the product's design and performance.

PHASE 3: REALIZE [MANUFACTURE, MAKE, BUILD, PROCURE, PRODUCE, SELL AND DELIVER]

Once the design of the product's components is complete, the method of manufacturing is defined. This phase involves creating computer numerical control (CNC) machining instructions for the product's parts as well as tools to manufacture those parts, using integrated or separate computer-aided manufacturing (CAM) software. It also involves analysis tools for process simulation for operations such as casting, molding, and die press forming.

Once the manufacturing method has been identified, Computer-Aided Process Planning (CAPP) comes into play. This involves the use of CAPE (Computer-Aided Production Engineering) or production planning tools for carrying out factory, plant, and facility layout and production simulation.

Other activities in this phase include procurement of raw materials, production scheduling, production control, and quality assurance. This is also the phase where the finished products are sold and delivered to customers.

PHASE 4: SERVICE [USE, OPERATE, MAINTAIN, SUPPORT, SUSTAIN, PHASE-OUT, RETIRE, RECYCLE AND DISPOSAL]

In the final phase of PLM, the product is already in the market and is being used by customers. The focus shifts to managing the product during its service life, including maintenance, support, and end-of-life considerations. Here are some of the activities involved in this phase:

1. ***Use and operate*:** This involves providing customers with user manuals, training, and other resources to help them use the product effectively.
2. ***Maintain and support*:** This includes providing support for the product, such as repairing or replacing parts, troubleshooting issues, and providing software updates or patches.
3. ***Sustain*:** The product needs to be sustained during its service life, which includes ensuring that it continues to meet customer needs, is up-to-date with current technology, and complies with regulatory requirements.
4. ***Phase-out and retire*:** As the product nears the end of its service life, it may be phased out or retired. This involves managing inventory levels, providing end-of-life support, and ensuring that customers have a smooth transition to a replacement product.
5. ***Recycle and disposal*:** Once the product has reached the end of its life, it must be disposed of or recycled in an environmentally responsible way. This involves managing the disposal process, ensuring compliance with regulations, and minimizing the environmental impact of the product.

Overall, the service phase of PLM is focused on ensuring that the product is a success throughout its entire life cycle, from design to retirement. By managing the product effectively during this phase, companies can improve customer satisfaction, reduce costs, and minimize environmental impact.

What is an FDA Inspection and why is it Necessary?

An FDA inspection is an on-site evaluation of a regulated facility or process to determine compliance with applicable laws and regulations. The FDA, or the Food and Drug Administration, is a federal agency of the United States Department of Health and Human Services that is responsible for regulating and supervising the safety and effectiveness of food, drugs, medical devices, and other products.

An FDA inspection is necessary to ensure that regulated products are safe, effective, and of high quality. The inspection process includes an evaluation of manufacturing processes, quality control procedures, laboratory methods, documentation practices, and other aspects of a regulated facility or process. The FDA may also review records, interview personnel, and collect samples during an inspection.

If the FDA finds that a facility or process is not in compliance with applicable laws and regulations, it may take enforcement actions, such as issuing a warning letter, initiating a recall, or seizing products. Therefore, an FDA inspection is an important tool for ensuring public health and safety.

Types of FDA Inspections

The FDA conducts various types of inspections to ensure compliance with regulations and standards. Some of the common types of FDA inspections are:

1. ***Pre-Approval Inspection (PAI)*:** Conducted before the approval of a new drug, medical device, or biologic product. The PAI focuses on the manufacturing process, facilities, and controls to ensure that they meet the FDA's standards.
2. ***Routine/Periodic Inspection*:** Conducted periodically to assess the compliance of the facility with the FDA's regulations and standards.
3. ***For-Cause Inspection*:** Conducted in response to a specific issue or concern, such as a product recall, adverse event, or complaint.
4. ***Follow-Up Inspection*:** Conducted to evaluate the corrective actions taken by a facility after a previous inspection.
5. ***Compliance/Mission Inspection*:** Conducted to assess a facility's overall compliance with FDA regulations and standards.
6. ***Surveillance Inspection*:** Conducted to monitor facilities that have had previous compliance issues to ensure that corrective actions are being taken and maintained.
7. ***Import Inspection*:** Conducted to inspect imported products to ensure they meet FDA regulations and standards.

8. ***Investigation Inspection*:** Conducted as part of an investigation into potential violations of FDA regulations and standards.
9. ***Team Biologics Inspection*:** Conducted to evaluate a facility's compliance with biologics regulations and standards.
10. ***Veterinary Medicine Inspection*:** Conducted to assess compliance with FDA regulations and standards related to animal drugs and devices.

FDA Inspector will verify:

During an FDA inspection, the FDA inspector will typically verify compliance with regulations related to the specific product or process being inspected. Some of the areas that the inspector may focus on include:

1. Manufacturing processes and procedures
2. Laboratory testing methods and procedures
3. Record-keeping and documentation practices
4. Facility cleanliness and sanitation
5. Adherence to Good Manufacturing Practices (GMPs)
6. Adequate product labeling and packaging
7. Adequate employee training and education
8. Quality control procedures and practices
9. Adequate testing and validation of equipment and processes
10. Complaint handling and adverse event reporting procedures.
11. The FDA inspector will review documents, observe manufacturing or testing processes, and interview employees to assess compliance with FDA regulations. The inspector may also take product samples for testing or request additional documentation or information.

Inspected documents

During an FDA inspection, the inspector will review a wide range of documents to ensure compliance with regulations and standards. Some of the commonly inspected documents may include:

1. Quality management system documents such as standard operating procedures (SOPs), work instructions, quality manuals, and policies.
2. Batch records and device history records (DHRs) for finished products, including labeling and packaging records.
3. Design history files (DHF) for medical devices, including design control documents and risk management plans.
4. Laboratory records, including test methods, specifications, and validation protocols and reports.

5. Manufacturing records, including equipment maintenance logs, calibration records, and cleaning records.
6. Complaint files, including customer complaints, investigation reports, and corrective and preventive action (CAPA) records.
7. Supplier qualification and management records, including supplier audits and performance records.
8. Training records, including employee training records and documentation for continuing education.
9. Import/export records, including customs documentation and bills of lading.
10. Adverse event and product defect reports, including medical device reports (MDRs) and field safety corrective action (FSCA) reports.

The FDA inspector will verify the accuracy, completeness, and adequacy of these documents and may request additional information or clarification as needed.

EIR: Establishment Investigation Report

In an Establishment Investigation Report (EIR), the inspector will typically review subject data to verify that:

1. ***The data is complete and accurate*:** The inspector will check that all required data has been collected and that it is accurate and reliable. They may also compare the data to previous records to ensure consistency.
2. ***The data meets regulatory requirements*:** The inspector will review the data to ensure that it meets the relevant regulatory requirements. This may include checking that the data was collected by standard operating procedures (SOPs) and that it complies with good manufacturing practices (GMPs).
3. ***The data supports the conclusions drawn*:** The inspector will evaluate the data to ensure that it supports the conclusions that were drawn based on the data. This may involve checking that the data analysis is appropriate and that any statistical methods used are valid.
4. ***The data is properly documented*:** The inspector will review the documentation associated with the data to ensure that it is complete and accurate. This may include checking that the data was properly recorded, that any deviations were appropriately documented, and that any changes to the data were properly authorized.

Overall, the inspector's goal in reviewing subject data is to ensure that it is reliable and accurate and that it supports the conclusions drawn in the EIR.

Warning Letter

A Warning Letter is a formal notice issued by the FDA to a company or individual who has violated FDA regulations. It is a serious enforcement action that indicates that the FDA has found significant violations of the Federal Food, Drug, and Cosmetic Act (the Act) or other FDA regulations.

The purpose of a Warning Letter is to notify the recipient of the violations and to request that they take prompt action to correct them. The letter will typically outline the specific violations that were identified during the FDA inspection, and it may include a list of corrective actions that the recipient is required to take.

If a company or individual does not take adequate corrective action in response to a Warning Letter, the FDA may take further enforcement action, which could include seizure of products, injunctions, or criminal prosecution.

Receiving a Warning Letter can have serious consequences for a company or individual, including damage to their reputation and financial losses. As such, it is important for companies to take FDA regulations seriously and to take prompt action to address any violations that are identified.

In addition to the immediate action required to address the violations outlined in the letter, a company may also face additional consequences, such as:

- ***Influence on approval*:** The FDA may withhold authorization for one or more of the company's products, or may not process pending applications.
- ***Import Stop/FDA Import Alert*:** The FDA may place an Import Alert on the company's products, which could prevent them from being imported into the United States.
- ***Court - Consent*:** The company may be required to undergo a consulting process to improve its systems and processes, which can be a time-consuming and costly endeavor.
- ***Seizure*:** The FDA may take legal action to remove violative goods from commerce by seizing them.
- ***Injunction*:** The FDA may seek a court order to prevent the company from violating or causing violations of the Act.
- ***Criminal prosecution*:** In cases where there is evidence of intent to violate the Act, the FDA may recommend criminal prosecution, which could result in fines and/or imprisonment for the responsible individuals.

It's important for companies to take FDA regulations seriously and to take prompt action to address any violations that are identified during an inspection, to avoid these potentially serious consequences.

Criminal Fines for Food Drug and Cosmetic Act Violations

Criminal fines for violations of the Food Drug and Cosmetic Act can be significant, and may depend on the severity of the violation and whether it is classified as a misdemeanor or felony.

For a misdemeanor violation, fines can range up to $100,000 for individuals and up to $200,000 for organizations. In addition, individuals may face imprisonment for up to one year.

For a felony violation, fines can range up to $250,000 for individuals and up to $500,000 for organizations. Individuals may face imprisonment for up to three years.

It's important to note that fines and penalties can vary based on the specific circumstances of the violation and that criminal fines are just one potential consequence of violating the Food Drug and Cosmetic Act. Companies may also face civil penalties, product seizures, import bans, and other regulatory actions. Therefore, it is essential for companies to prioritize compliance with FDA regulations and to take prompt action to address any violations that are identified during an inspection.

Establishment Inspection Report

An Establishment Inspection Report (EIR) is a document that summarizes the findings of an FDA inspection of a regulated establishment, such as a pharmaceutical or medical device manufacturer, food processor, or cosmetic manufacturer. The EIR is prepared by the FDA investigator who conducted the inspection and provides a detailed account of any deficiencies or violations observed during the inspection.

The EIR includes information on the facility, such as the name and location, as well as details about the inspection process, such as the date of the inspection and the length of time it took. It also includes a summary of the observations made by the investigator, including any deficiencies or violations that were identified. The report may also include observations on the quality control and quality assurance procedures, documentation practices, and any corrective actions taken by the establishment during the inspection.

The EIR is an important document that is used by the FDA to evaluate the compliance of regulated establishments with FDA regulations and to determine the appropriate regulatory action to take if deficiencies or violations are identified. Depending on the nature and severity of the deficiencies or violations identified during the inspection, the FDA may take a range of regulatory actions, including issuing a warning letter, imposing fines or other penalties, or even seeking criminal prosecution.

Establishment Inspection Report

An Establishment Inspection Report (EIR) is a report generated by FDA inspectors after inspecting a regulated establishment. The EIR contains details of the inspection findings, compliance status, and any corrective actions taken or recommended. The following are some key components of an EIR:

1. ***Establishment Information*:** The EIR should include basic information about the establishment that was inspected, such as the name, address, and type of establishment.
2. ***Inspection Details*:** The EIR should provide details about the inspection, such as the dates of the inspection, the names of the FDA inspectors, and the areas of the establishment that were inspected.
3. ***Observations*:** The EIR should contain a detailed account of the observations made during the inspection, including any deficiencies or violations identified.
4. ***Compliance Status*:** The EIR should indicate the compliance status of the establishment, including any areas of non-compliance that were identified during the inspection.
5. ***Corrective Actions*:** The EIR should describe any corrective actions taken by the establishment to address the deficiencies or violations identified during the inspection.
6. ***Recommendations*:** The EIR should include recommendations for further improvements or corrective actions, if necessary.
7. ***Conclusion*:** The EIR should conclude with a summary of the inspection findings, compliance status, and any recommendations for further action.

Overall, an EIR is an important document that helps to ensure the safety and quality of regulated products. It serves as a record of the inspection findings and helps to ensure that establishments comply with FDA regulations.

A good inspection visit report must contain the following information:

A good inspection visit report should contain the following information:

1. ***Background Information*:** This should include basic information about the establishment, such as the name, location, and type of business.
2. ***Scope of Inspection*:** This should outline the areas of the establishment that were inspected and the purpose of the inspection.
3. ***Inspection Findings*:** This should provide a detailed account of the inspection findings, including any observations made, deficiencies or violations identified, and any corrective actions taken or recommended.
4. ***Compliance Status*:** This should indicate the compliance status of the establishment, including any areas of non-compliance that were identified during the inspection.

5. ***Follow-Up Action***: This should outline any follow-up action that is required, including corrective actions to be taken by the establishment, any re-inspection requirements, and any deadlines for compliance.
6. ***Conclusion***: This should summarize the inspection findings and provide an overall assessment of the establishment's compliance status.
7. ***Appendices***: This should include any additional information that supports the inspection findings, such as photographs, test results, or other documentation.

In general, a good inspection visit report should be thorough, well-organized, and easy to understand. It should provide a clear assessment of the establishment's compliance status and any actions that are required to ensure compliance with regulatory requirements.

Establishment Inspection Report- Release Note

A release note is a document that accompanies the Establishment Inspection Report (EIR) when it is released to the inspected establishment. The release note provides a summary of the inspection findings and outlines any follow-up action that is required. The release note typically includes the following information:

1. ***Inspection Findings***: A summary of the inspection findings, including any observations made, deficiencies or violations identified, and any corrective actions taken or recommended.
2. ***Compliance Status***: A clear indication of the compliance status of the establishment, including any areas of non-compliance that were identified during the inspection.
3. ***Follow-Up Action***: An outline of any follow-up action that is required, including corrective actions to be taken by the establishment, any re-inspection requirements, and any deadlines for compliance.
4. ***Conclusion***: A summary of the inspection findings and an overall assessment of the establishment's compliance status.

The release note is an important document that helps to ensure that the inspected establishment is aware of the inspection findings and any follow-up action that is required. The release note must be clear and easy to understand, so that the establishment can take appropriate action to address any areas of non-compliance.

Recall

Recall refers to the process of removing or correcting products that are deemed to be unsafe, defective, or otherwise in violation of regulatory standards. Recalls can be initiated by the manufacturer, importer, or distributor of a product, or by a regulatory agency such as the FDA.

Recalls can be voluntary or mandatory, depending on the circumstances. In a voluntary recall, the manufacturer, importer, or distributor initiates the recall on their own accord. In a mandatory recall, the regulatory agency requires the recall to be conducted.

Recalls can be initiated for a variety of reasons, such as:

- Contamination with harmful substances
- Presence of undeclared allergens
- Defective or malfunctioning products
- Mislabeling or misbranding
- Failure to meet regulatory standards

Recalls can have significant financial and reputational impacts on the company involved. Companies need to have effective quality control and risk management systems in place to minimize the risk of recalls, and to have plans in place for handling recalls if they do occur.

Seizure and Injunction

Seizure and injunction are two different types of enforcement actions that the FDA can take against regulated products or companies that violate the Federal Food, Drug, and Cosmetic Act.

Seizure is an action brought against an FDA-regulated product because it is adulterated and/or misbranded within the meaning of the Act. The purpose of such an action is to remove specific violative goods from commerce. If the FDA determines that a product is in violation of the Act and poses a threat to public health, it can initiate a seizure action to remove the product from the market. The FDA can seize products that are adulterated or misbranded, and the seizure can occur at any point in the distribution chain, including at the manufacturer, distributor, or retailer level.

The injunction, on the other hand, is an order by a court that requires an individual or corporation to do or refrain from doing a specific act. The FDA may seek injunctions against individuals and/or corporations to prevent them from violating or causing violations of the Act. For example, the FDA may seek an injunction against a company that is continuing to manufacture and distribute a product that violates the Act. Injunctions can be temporary or permanent and can be issued by a court after a trial or as part of a settlement agreement.

Both seizure and injunction are serious enforcement actions that can have significant consequences for regulated companies, including the loss of business and damage to reputation. The FDA considers a range of factors when deciding whether to take these actions, including the nature and severity of the violation, the potential harm to public health, and the company's compliance history.

ISO Risk Management Standard

ISO 31000 is an international standard for risk management. It provides principles, a framework, and a process for managing risk effectively. The standard was first published in 2009 and revised in 2018.

The standard applies to any organization, regardless of its size, type, or nature. It provides a common approach to managing risks that can be applied across different sectors and industries.

The ISO 31000 risk management standard is based on the following principles:

1. Risk management creates and protects value.
2. Risk management is an integral part of all organizational processes.
3. Risk management is part of decision-making.
4. Risk management explicitly addresses uncertainty.
5. Risk management is systematic, structured, and timely.
6. Risk management is based on the best available information.
7. Risk management is tailored.
8. Risk management takes into account human and cultural factors.
9. Risk management is transparent and inclusive.
10. Risk management is dynamic, iterative, and responsive to change.

The standard provides a framework for managing risk that includes:

1. Establishing the context for risk management, including defining the scope, criteria, and objectives.
2. Risk assessment, including identifying, analyzing, and evaluating risks.
3. Risk treatment, including selecting and implementing risk treatment options.
4. Risk communication and consultation, including sharing information about risks and involving stakeholders in the risk management process.
5. Monitoring and review, including reviewing and continuously improving the risk management process.

ISO 31000 is a voluntary standard and is not intended for certification purposes. However, organizations can use the standard as a basis for developing their risk management frameworks and processes.

Practice Questions

MCQs

1. Product lifecycle management (LCM) is the process of managing the entire lifecycle of a product including its research, design and manufacture, service, and disposal.

   a. True   b. False

2. Product lifecycle management should include

   a. new indications
   b. improved formulation
   c. new delivery system, IT solutions,
   d. All of the above

3. What Types of Safety Labeling Changes Could Be Required Under Section 505(o)(4)

   a. Boxed warnings   b. Drug interactions
   c. Adverse reactions   d. All of the above

4. How many phases of product lifecycle management include

   a. 5   b. 4
   c. 3   d. 2

5. Which of the following are product lifecycle management benefits

   a. framework for product optimization
   b. Reduced prototyping costs
   c. Ability to quickly identify potential sales opportunities and revenue contributions
   d. All of the above

6. EIR stands for

   a. Establishment Investigation Report
   b. Establishment Invest Report
   c. Establish Investigation Report
   d. Establishment Improvement Report

7. Prescription drug products with an approved new drug application (NDA) under section 505(b) of the Act

   a. True   b. False

8. Prescription drug products with an approved new drug application (NDA) under section 505(b) of the Act.

   a. True
   b. False

Short Answer Questions

Q.1 Short note on Post approval changes.

Q.2 Explain Warning letters and recall.

Q.3 Short note on the establishment investigation report.

Long Answer Questions

Q.1. Explain prior approval and post-approval changes supplement.

Q.2. Outline the process of prior approval supplement (PAS), post-approval changes and CBE-30.

Answers to MCQs

1. a	2. d	3. d	4. b
5. d	6. a	7. a	8. a

References

1. Compliance auditing for Pharmaceutical Manufacturers. Karen Ginsbury and Gil Bismuth, Interpharm/CRC, Boca Raton, London NewYork, Washington D.C.

2. Pharmaceutical Manufacturing Handbook, Regulations and Quality by Shayne Cox Gad. Wiley-Interscience, A John Wiley and sons, Inc., Publications.

3. Handbook of microbiological Quality control. Rosamund M. Baird, Norman A. Hodges, Stephen P. Denyar. CRC Press. 2000.

4. Laboratory auditing for quality and regulatory compliance. Donald C. Singer, Raluca-loana Stefan, Jacobus F. Van Staden. Taylor and Francis (2005).

5. Implementing Juran's Road Map for Quality Leadership: Benchmarks and Results, By Al Endres, Wiley, 2000

6. Understanding, Managing and Implementing Quality: Frameworks, Techniques and Cases, By Jiju Antony; David Preece, Routledge, 2002

7. Organizing for High Performance: Employee Involvement, TQM, Reengineering, and Knowledge Management in the Fortune 1000: The CEO Report By Edward E. Lawler; Susan Albers Mohrman; George Benson, Jossey-Bass, 2001

8. Corporate Culture and the Quality Organization By James W. FairfieldSonn, Quorum Books, 2001

9. The Quality Management Sourcebook: An International Guide to Materials and Resources By Christine Avery; Diane Zabel, Routledge, 1997

10. The Quality Toolbox, Second Edition, Nancy R. Tague, ASQPublicationsPills, Paper Planes, December 16, 2019, https://www.joinpaperplanes.com

www.ingramcontent.com/pod-product-compliance
Ingram Content Group UK Ltd.
Pitfield, Milton Keynes, MK11 3LW, UK
UKHW020047200726
13845UKWH00044B/12

9 789349 562479